Respiratory and Cardiac Gating in PET Imaging

Editors

HABIB ZAIDI
B. KEVIN TEO

PET CLINICS

www.pet.theclinics.com

Consulting Editor
ABASS ALAVI

January 2013 • Volume 8 • Number 1

ELSEVIER

1600 John F. Kennedy Boulevard • Suite 1800 • Philadelphia, Pennsylvania 19103-2899

http://www.theclinics.com

PET CLINICS Volume 8, Number 1
January 2013 ISSN 1556-8598, ISBN-13: 978-1-4557-7138-7

Editor: Adrianne Brigido

PET Clinics (ISSN 1556-8598) is published quarterly by Elsevier Inc., 360 Park Avenue South, New York, NY 10010-1710. Months of issue are January, April, July, and October. Periodicals postage paid at New York, NY, and additional mailing offices. Subscription prices per year are $215.00 (US individuals), $297.00 (US institutions), $110.00 (US students), $244.00 (Canadian individuals), $332.00 (Canadian institutions), $124.00 (Canadian students), $260.00 (foreign individuals), $332.00 (foreign institutions), and $134.00 (foreign students). To receive student and resident rate, orders must be accompanied by name of affiliated institution, date of term, and the signature of program/residency coordinator on institution letterhead. Orders will be billed at individual rate until proof of status is received. Foreign air speed delivery is included in all Clinics subscription prices. All prices are subject to change without notice. POSTMASTER: Send address changes to PET Clinics, Elsevier Health Sciences Division, Subscription Customer Service, 3251 Riverport Lane, Maryland Heights, MO 63043. **Customer Service: 1-800-654-2452 (U.S. and Canada); 314-447-8871 (outside U.S. and Canada). Fax: 314-447-8029. E-mail: journalscustomerservice-usa@elsevier.com (for print support); journalsonlinesupport-usa@elsevier.com (for online support).**

Reprints. For copies of 100 or more of articles in this publication, please contact the Commercial Reprints Department, Elsevier Inc., 360 Park Avenue South, New York, NY 10010-1710. Tel.: 212-633-3812; Fax: 212-462-1935; E-mail: reprints@elsevier.com.

Printed in the United States of America.

Contributors

CONSULTING EDITOR

ABASS ALAVI, MD, PhD (Hon), DSc (Hon)
Professor of Radiology, Division of Nuclear
Medicine, University of Pennsylvania School of
Medicine; Department of Radiology, Hospital
of the University of Pennsylvania, Philadelphia,
Pennsylvania

GUEST EDITORS

HABIB ZAIDI, PhD, PD
Division of Nuclear Medicine and Molecular
Imaging, Geneva University Hospital; Geneva
Neuroscience Center, Geneva University,
Geneva, Switzerland; Department of Nuclear
Medicine and Molecular Imaging, University
Medical Center Groningen, University of
Groningen, Groningen, Netherlands

B. KEVIN TEO, PhD
Department of Radiation Oncology, University
of Pennsylvania, Philadelphia, Pennsylvania

AUTHORS

V. BETTINARDI, MSc
Department of Nuclear Medicine, Ospedale
San Raffaele; IBFM-CNR, Institute for
Molecular Bioimaging and Physiology,
Segrate, Milano, Italy

RALPH A. BUNDSCHUH, PhD
Klinik und Poliklinik für Nuklearmedizin,
Universitätsklinikum Würzburg, München,
Germany

LAURENCE E. COURT, PhD
Assistant Professor, Departments of Radiation
and Imaging Physics, The University of
Texas MD Anderson Cancer Center,
Houston, Texas

E. DE BERNARDI, PhD
Department of Nuclear Medicine, Ospedale
San Raffaele, Segrate, Milano, Italy;
Department of Health Sciences; TECNOMED
Foundation, University of Milano-Bicocca,
Monza, Italy

JULIA DINGES, MD
Klinik und Poliklinik für Nuklearmedizin,
Klinikum rechts der Isar der Technischen
Universität München; Nuklearmedizinische
Klinik und Poliklinik der Technischen
Universität München, München, Germany

ANASTASIOS GAITANIS, MSc, PhD
Department of Biomedical Technology,
Biomedical Research Foundation of the
Academy of Athens, Athens, Greece

M.C. GILARDI, MSc
Department of Nuclear Medicine, Ospedale
San Raffaele; IBFM-CNR, Institute for
Molecular Bioimaging and Physiology,
Segrate, Milano, Italy; Department of Health
Sciences; TECNOMED Foundation, University
of Milano-Bicocca, Monza, Italy

OSAMA R. MAWLAWI, PhD
Professor, Department of Imaging Physics, The
University of Texas MD Anderson Cancer
Center, Houston, Texas

SADEK A. NEHMEH, PhD
Department of Medical Physics, Memorial Sloan-Kettering Cancer Center, New York, New York

STEPHAN G. NEKOLLA, PhD
Klinik und Poliklinik für Nuklearmedizin, Klinikum rechts der Isar der Technischen Universität München; Nuklearmedizinische Klinik der Technischen Universität München, München, Germany

TINSU PAN, PhD
Department of Imaging Physics, MD Anderson Cancer Center, The University of Texas, Houston, Texas

L. PRESOTTO, MSc
Department of Nuclear Medicine, Ospedale San Raffaele, Segrate, Milano, Italy; Department of Physics G. Occhialini, University of Milano Bicocca, Milano, Italy

ARMAN RAHMIM, PhD
Division of Nuclear Medicine, Department of Radiology, Johns Hopkins University, Baltimore, Maryland

CHRISTOPH RISCHPLER, MD
Nuklearmedizinische Klinik und Poliklinik der Technischen Universität München, München, Germany

JING TANG, PhD
Department of Electrical and Computer Engineering, Oakland University, Rochester, Michigan

CHARALAMPOS TSOUMPAS, MPhys, MSc, DIC, PhD
Division of Imaging Sciences and Biomedical Engineering, Department of Biomedical Engineering, King's College London, King's Health Partners, St. Thomas' Hospital, London, United Kingdom

HABIB ZAIDI, PhD, PD
Division of Nuclear Medicine and Molecular Imaging, Geneva University Hospital; Geneva Neuroscience Center, Geneva University, Geneva, Switzerland; Department of Nuclear Medicine and Molecular Imaging, University Medical Center Groningen, University of Groningen, Groningen, Netherlands

Contents

Image quality in PET examinations is influenced by several factors. Patient motion during PET data acquisition is a substantial problem that potentially leads to smearing artifacts, resulting in the loss of diagnostic accuracy both in visual and quantitative image analyses. In hybrid imaging, coregistration of functional (PET) and morphologic (CT or MR imaging) data can be hampered by patient movement between the acquisitions, resulting in additional sources of error. This article describes the artifacts due to patient movement.

Respiratory and cardiac motions represent important sources of image degradation in both PET and computed tomography (CT) studies that need to be taken into account and compensated to improve image quality and quantitative accuracy. This review describes the hardware needed to perform respiratory and cardiac gating with PET and PET/CT systems. In particular, most of the proposed motion-tracking devices for the management of respiratory, cardiac, and multidimensional movements are described and compared. Some advanced applications in PET and PET/CT made possible by the gating technology are considered and analyzed.

PET-CT scanners allow robust and synergistic fusion of anatomic and functional information, which has improved sensitivity, specificity, and enhancement in the value of PET and CT when assessing tumor response to therapy. Breathing motion and the difference in time resolutions commonly cause motion artifacts and spatial mismatch between the corresponding image sets. Correction for the breathing-induced artifacts represents a particular challenge. This article summarizes the materials, methods, and results involved in multiple investigations of the correction for respiratory motion in PET-CT imaging of the thorax. Some methods use respiratory-phase data selection, whereas others have adopted sophisticated software techniques.

This article discusses attenuation correction strategies in positron emission tomography/computed tomography (PET/CT) and 4-dimensional PET/CT imaging. Average CT scan derived from averaging the high temporal resolution CT images is effective in improving the registration of the CT and the PET images and quantification of the PET data. It underscores list-mode data acquisition in 4-dimensional PET, and introduces 4-dimensional CT, popular in thoracic treatment planning, to 4-dimensional PET/CT.

Cardiac and respiratory movements pose significant challenges to image quality and quantitative accuracy in PET imaging. Cardiac and/or respiratory gating attempt to address this issue, but instead lead to enhanced noise levels. Direct four-dimensional (4D) PET image reconstruction incorporating motion compensation has the potential to minimize noise amplification while removing considerable motion blur. A wide-ranging choice of such techniques is reviewed in this work. Future opportunities and the challenges facing the adoption of 4D PET reconstruction and its role in basic and clinical research are also discussed.

Electrocardiogram-gated cardiac positron emission tomography is a valuable addition to the armamentarium of clinical positron emission tomography. It provides incremental diagnostic information and can be conveniently embedded into clinical protocols. In the same way electrocardiogram gating was added to myocardial perfusion single photon emission computed tomography, it can be expected that this approach will be a standard component in the future.

Radiation oncology has evolved to the point at which it is ripe for the clinical introduction of routine four-dimensional (4D) PET-CT scanning. The initial use of 4D PET-CT will be for target definition, followed by the use of standardized uptake values (SUVs) for dose-painting. 4D PET-CT also has some potential applications in outcome prediction and dose-response studies.

The driving force in the research and development of new hybrid PET-CT/MR imaging scanners is the production of images with optimum quality, accuracy, and resolution. However, the acquisition process is limited by several factors. Key issues are the respiratory and cardiac motion artifacts that occur during an imaging session. In this article the necessary tools for modeling and simulation of realistic high-resolution four-dimensional PET-CT and PET-MR imaging data are described. Beyond the need for four-dimensional simulations, accurate modeling of the acquisition process can be included within the reconstruction algorithms assisting in the improvement of image quality and accuracy of estimation of physiologic parameters from four-dimensional hybrid PET imaging.

PET CLINICS

PROGRAM OBJECTIVE:

The goal of the PET Clinics of North America is to keep practicing radiologists and radiology residents up to date with current clinical practice in positron emission tomography by providing timely articles reviewing the state of the art in patient care.

TARGET AUDIENCE

All practicing physicians and healthcare professionals who provide patient care utilizing findings from *Positron Emission Tomography Clinics of North America*.

ACCREDITATION

The Elsevier Office of Continuing Medical Education (EOCME) is accredited by the Accreditation Council for Continuing Medical Education (ACCME) to provide continuing medical education for physicians.

The EOCME designates this journal-based CME activity for a maximum of 8 *AMA PRA Category 1 Credit*(s)™. Physicians should claim only the credit commensurate with the extent of their participation in the activity.

All other health care professionals completing continuing education credit for this activity will be issued a certificate of participation.

DISCLOSURE OF CONFLICTS OF INTEREST

The EOCME assesses conflict of interest with its instructors, faculty, planners, and other individuals who are in a position to control the content of CME activities. All relevant conflicts of interest that are identified are thoroughly vetted by EOCME for fair balance, scientific objectivity, and patient care recommendations. EOCME is committed to providing its learners with CME activities that promote improvements or quality in healthcare and not a specific proprietary business or a commercial interest.

The planning committee, staff, authors and editors listed below have identified no financial relationships or relationships to products or devices they or their spouse/life partner have with commercial interest related to the content of this CME activity:

V. Bettinardi, MSc; Laurence E. Court, PhD; E. De Bernardi, PhD; Anastasios Gaitanis, MSc, PhD; M.C. Gilardi, MSc; Osama R. Mawlawi, PhD; Jill McNair; Sadek A. Nehmeh, PhD; Stephan G. Nekolla, PhD; L. Presotto, MSc; Arman Rahmim, PhD; Christoph Rischpler, MD; Katelynn Steck; Jing Tang, PhD; B. Kevin Teo, PhD; Charalampos Tsoumpas, MPhys, MSc, DIC, PhD; and Habib Zaidi, PhD, PD.

The planning committee, staff, authors and editors listed below have identified financial relationships or relationships to products or devices they or their spouse/life partner have with commercial interest related to the content of this CME activity:

Ralph A. Bundschuh, PhD has received research funding from Mediso Medical Imaging Systems.
Julia Dinges, MD has received research funding from Mediso Medical Imaging Systems.
Tinsu Pan, PhD owns stock in Texas Medical Imaging Consultants, LLC.

UNAPPROVED/OFF-LABEL USE DISCLOSURE

The EOCME requires CME faculty to disclose to the participants:

1. When products or procedures being discussed are off-label, unlabelled, experimental, and/or investigational (not US Food and Drug Administration (FDA) approved; and
2. Any limitations on the information presented, such as data that are preliminary or that represent ongoing research, interim analyses, and/or unsupported opinions. Faculty may discuss information about pharmaceutical agents that is outside of DA-approved labelling. This information is intended solely for CME and is not intended to promote off-label use of these medications. If you have any questions, contact the medical affairs department of the manufacturer for the most recent prescribing information.

TO ENROLL

To enroll in the PET Clinics Continuing Medical Education program, call customer service at 1-800-654-2452 or sign up online at http://www.theclinics.com/home/cme. The CME program is available to subscribers for an additional annual fee of $212 USD.

METHOD OF PARTICIPATION

In order to claim credit, participants must complete the following:

1. Complete enrolment as indicated above.
2. Read the activity.
3. Complete the CME Test and Evaluation. Participants must achieve a score of 70% on the test. All CME Tests and Evaluations must be completed online.

CME INQUIRIES/SPECIAL NEEDS

For all CME inquiries or special needs, please contact elsevierCME@elsevier.com.

Preface

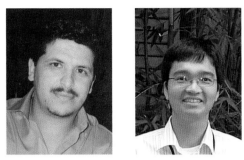

Habib Zaidi, PhD, PD   B. Kevin Teo, PhD
Guest Editors

In the era of molecular imaging,[1] positron emission tomography (PET) and single-photon emission computed tomography using highly specific probes have enabled biomedical researchers to study biochemical processes at the molecular level. The rapid pace in the development of emission tomography imaging technology has been motivated by the desire of clinicians and biomedical imaging researchers to produce ever more detailed and quantitatively accurate images for diagnosis, staging, therapy response monitoring, and radiation therapy treatment planning. This drive has led the academic community as well as commercial vendors to develop new molecular agents, detector technologies, image reconstruction algorithms, and data processing software. The integration of PET and CT in a single gantry has enabled better localization of metabolic abnormalities, which in turn spurred the need to further improve PET sensitivity, image resolution, and quantification. While PET scanner sensitivity and image resolution can be improved by new detector technologies, correcting for motion blurring requires a fundamentally different approach.

Motion is a particularly challenging problem in PET. Respiratory motion in the thoracic and abdominal regions can be up to several centimeters and results in a smeared image with reduced quantification accuracy. The effect of motion can be further compounded by errors in attenuation correction that may lead to a wrong diagnosis. For cardiac applications, both respiratory and cardiac motion lead to image artefacts that affect diagnosis. In recent years, gating techniques were developed for PET/CT imaging to reduce motion artefacts. While some level of success has been achieved with these gating techniques, there is still room for further improvement. In particular, the issue of reduced signal-to-noise ratio, irregular breathing motion, and accuracy of external motion surrogate must be addressed. With the development of PET/MRI systems[2,3] capable of simultaneous acquisition, highly advanced non-rigid motion correction strategies are becoming possible.[4] While this technology is still in its infancy, it is a promising development that seems to have the potential to overcome all the deficiencies with current gating techniques. Further exciting developments in technology to address motion lie ahead for researchers in this field.

This issue of *PET Clinics* addresses the subject of gating in PET as a method to reduce motion artefacts and discusses the hardware and software tools available. As the use of gating becomes more widespread, its role and limitations in the clinical setting for clinical oncology and cardiology applications are being debated. Advanced topics related to gating, such as computer modeling and simulation, are also discussed. It is hoped that this collection of comprehensive topics in gating will serve as instructional information for readers interested in understanding current gating technology and its applications.

PET Clin 8 (2013) ix–x
http://dx.doi.org/10.1016/j.cpet.2012.10.006
1556-8598/13/$ – see front matter Published by Elsevier Inc.

Habib Zaidi, PhD, PD
Division of Nuclear Medicine
and Molecular Imaging
Geneva University Hospital
CH-1211 Geneva, Switzerland

B. Kevin Teo, PhD
Department of Radiation Oncology
University of Pennsylvania
Philadelphia, PA 19104, USA

E-mail addresses:
habib.zaidi@hcuge.ch (H. Zaidi)
kevin.teo@uphs.upenn.edu (B.K. Teo)

REFERENCES

1. Gambhir SS. Molecular Imaging of cancer with positron emission tomography. Nat Rev Cancer 2002; 2(9):683–93.
2. Drzezga A, Souvatzoulou M, Eiber M, et al. First clinical experience with integrated whole-body PET/MR: Comparison to PET/CT in patients with oncologic diagnoses. J Nucl Med 2012;53:845–55.
3. Zaidi H, Del Guerra A. An outlook on future design of hybrid PET/MRI systems. Med Phys 2011;38(10):5667–89.
4. Chun SY, Reese TG, Ouyang J, et al. MRI-based nonrigid motion correction in simultaneous PET/MRI. J Nucl Med 2012;53:1284–91.

Motion Artifacts in Oncological and Cardiac PET Imaging

Julia Dinges, MD[a], Stephan G. Nekolla, PhD[a],
Ralph A. Bundschuh, PhD[b],*

KEYWORDS

- Motion artifacts • PET • Hybrid imaging • Respiratory motion • Cardiac motion

KEY POINTS

- Patient movement is the main limiting factor of PET/CT image quality.
- Respiratory and cardiac motion lead to smearing artifacts in PET images, resulting in errors in both qualitative and quantitative image analysis.
- In hybrid imaging, coregistration of functional and morphologic data can be complicated by patient movement and hence induce additional artifacts and errors, for example, in attenuation correction.

INTRODUCTION

Over the past years, PET has been established as a standard medical imaging modality, especially in oncology, cardiology, and neurology where PET imaging is frequently performed. Owing to the development of novel PET radiopharmaceuticals[1,2] as well as progress in hardware and software technology, for example, by introduction of point spread reconstruction[3] or time-of-flight PET,[4,5] image quality and hence diagnostic accuracy has improved significantly in recent years. But the high spatial resolution of modern PET machines has made a formerly minor concern become more and more important. Hence patient movement and organ motion is currently one of the main limiting factors of image quality in PET.

PET data acquisition can take several minutes and up to more than 1 hour, for example, studies for kinetic modeling. Owing to the long acquisition time, PET examinations are extremely sensitive to patient movement, which can cause reduced image quality and motion artifacts in the final images. Movement throughout data acquisition leads to smearing of active structures. Hence, borders of adjacent structures might not be clearly visible, leading to interpretation errors. In addition, smearing artifacts lead to false-low quantification of activity concentration and false-high volumes of active structures. Besides quantification errors, detection of small structures or lesions is complicated by a low signal-to-background ratio.

Since the introduction of integrated PET and computed tomography (PET/CT) systems in 2002,[6] functional and morphologic imaging is mostly combined these days. Anatomic information facilitates the localization of pathologic findings and also helps in discriminating pathologic and physiologic findings, for example, F18-fludeoxy-glucose (FDG) uptake in the bowel or in brown fat tissue.[7–9] However, new problems in imaging occur due to the integration of 2 completely different modalities. PET data acquisition takes several minutes and hence is an averaged image with respect to patient movement. In contrast, CT data are snap shots of one motion state due to the

Disclosure: All authors declare that there are no conflicts of interest to disclose within the context of this manuscript.
[a] Klinik und Poliklinik für Nuklearmedizin, Klinikum rechts der Isar der Technischen Universität München, Ismaninger Str. 22, München 81675, Germany; [b] Klinik und Poliklinik für Nuklearmedizin, Universitätsklinikum Würzburg, Oberdürrbacher Str. 6, München 97080, Germany
* Corresponding author.
E-mail address: ralph.bundschuh@gmx.de

acquisition time of several seconds. Thus, alignment of functional and morphologic data sets can be difficult and numerous artifacts may occur. In addition, misalignment of PET and CT images may cause errors in quantitative information of PET because CT is used as transmission data to correct the PET information for scatter and attenuation.[10]

Recently, integrated PET and magnetic resonance (MR) imaging systems were introduced.[11] There are 2 different technical solutions of combined PET/MR imaging machines. In the serial solution, the same patient table but a separate gantry is used for acquisition of PET and MR data for optimal coregistration and shorter examination times. As in PET/CT, such a serial design is more prone to motion inconsistencies between the functional and anatomic acquisitions. In the second solution, PET and MR imaging are integrated into the same gantry, providing the possibility of simultaneous data acquisition and reduction of misalignment of PET and MR imaging due to patient movement. However, to set up acquisition protocols for simultaneous acquisition of PET and MR imaging is technically demanding and additional work needs to be done in this field.

There are different sources of motion during PET acquisition: whole body movement occurs especially during long acquisition times and/or in patients with pain or any other kind of discomfort. In these cases, movement is easily detected from the image because it causes strong artifacts. Involuntary movement is caused by vegetative body processes, which cannot be directly controlled by the patient.

Two different types of involuntary movement can be distinguished: the nonperiodic movement, for example, changes in size and shape of internal organs such as during bowel movement or filling of the bladder, and the periodic movement, for example, respiration or heart beat. These periodic movements, especially respiration, are the main sources of motion artifacts in PET imaging because of continuous movement during data acquisition and no possibility of avoiding the movement.

The first section of this article will discuss motion artifacts appearing in oncological whole body imaging explained in examples. The second section will discuss special aspects of cardiac PET imaging.

MOTION ARTIFACTS
Oncological Imaging

In oncology, PET imaging is mainly used for diagnosis, staging, therapy planning, and therapy monitoring of malignant diseases. In tumor diagnosis and staging, the most important issue is to detect and localize pathologic tracer uptake. In therapy planning and monitoring of malignant diseases, quantification of lesion size and tracer uptake is the most important issue.

The signal-to-background ratio of a lesion is the most important factor for lesion detection. The higher the ratio, the easier it is to detect a pathologic uptake. Patient movement during data acquisition can lead to smearing of the PET images, as illustrated in **Fig. 1**, which decreases lesion signal intensity but does not affect the background activity, and hence the signal-to-background ratio

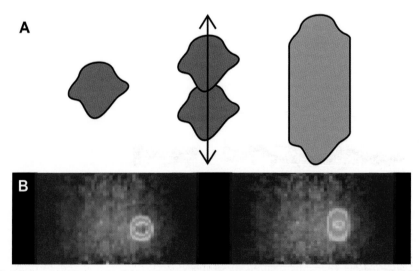

Fig. 1. (*A*) Illustration of a structure with positive uptake (*left*). Owing to periodic movement (*middle*), eg, respiration, uptake of the structure is smeared over a volume larger than the structure itself (*right*) resulting in an overestimation of the volume and an underestimation of the uptake. (*B*) PET image of a phantom sphere in background activity without (*left*) and with (*right*) movement (28 mm amplitude) of the sphere.

is reduced (**Fig. 2**). In contrast to whole body motion, which mainly occurs as a single event during data acquisition, periodic movement such as respiratory or cardiac motion causes blurring artifacts. When the heart contracts it does not affect adjacent structures but only itself. Hence cardiac motion, which will be discussed in the following section, is of importance only for cardiac imaging. In oncological imaging, respiratory motion is a big challenge. The largest motion artifacts can be seen in the thorax and the upper abdomen, showing an average movement of 13 mm of the liver and the spleen and of 11 mm of the kidneys.[12] However, maximum values of up to 50 mm (liver) and 40 mm (spleen) have been reported.[13] Depending on the location of lung tumors, lesions were found to move up to 18.5 mm because of respiration during PET imaging.[14] In MR imaging, tumor movement of up to 24 mm was found, especially in lesions of the lower lobes.[15] Even high spatial resolution of modern PET scanners of 5 to 7 mm is quite low compared to morphologic imaging such as CT or MR imaging. This motion extent can have remarkable effects on PET images.

Smearing artifacts not only reduce detectability of lesions but also alter quantitative accuracy of PET images. Owing to regular periodic movement during data acquisition, the tracer concentration in lesions seems to be reduced. In addition, the lesion seems larger in a smeared image than it is in reality (see **Fig. 1**). A study using a phantom with moveable spheres showed a difference in volume of 50% for a 23 mL hot sphere in background activity when simulating a motion amplitude of 28 mm. Consequently, an underestimation of the

activity concentration in the sphere of up to 14% was found.[14] The same study demonstrated a difference of lesion volume of up to 27% and of up to 13% of mean activity concentration on comparing PET signal with and without motion correction in patients with lung tumors.[14] Comparing respiratory corrected and uncorrected data, Nehmeh and colleagues[16] found a difference of lesion volume of 28% and of lesion uptake of 56.5% in one of their patients. Motion effects are especially important in PET studies performed for monitoring therapy response because these differences can have major influence in lesion uptake.[17,18] Thus, errors in image quantification due to patient movement may potentially lead to incorrect clinical decisions.

Recently, PET has also been established as an important tool in the planning of radiation therapy in several tumor sites, for example, lung[19] and brain tumors[20] as well as lymphoma.[21] Metabolic information provided by PET often allows an improved determination of vital tumor and adjacent tissue, for example, atelectasis[19] or scar tissue in previously treated patients.[22,23] In radiation treatment planning, estimation of the volume of the lesion is essential. Therefore, motion artifacts and the resulting errors in volume quantification can lead to severe overestimation of the lesion size. This overestimation may result in incorrect radiation field margins in the treatment plan, which delivers unnecessarily high radiation dose to the surrounding healthy tissue.

Patient motion can lead to artifacts that reduce detectability of small lesions and induce errors in quantification of tracer uptake and lesion size. In hybrid imaging, additional problems may appear.

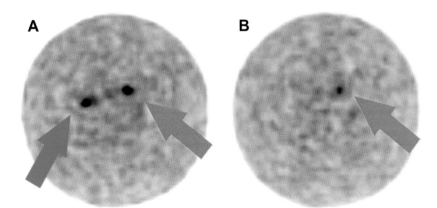

Fig. 2. Transaxial images of a 20-cm cylinder phantom including a 10-mm (*red arrow*) sphere and an 8-mm (*green arrow*) sphere. Background and spheres were filled with ^{18}F solution; the signal-to-background ratio was 7:1. (*A*) PET data were acquired without any movement of the spheres. While the 10-mm sphere is visible on both images, the signal-to-background ratio of the 8-mm sphere is too low because of motion blurring and is thus not visible in (*B*). (*B*) PET image acquisition was performed while the spheres were moved linearly in axial direction with an amplitude of 30 mm.

Owing to numerous advantages, PET examinations are at present mostly performed on integrated PET/CT devices. One of the advantages is a shorter acquisition time with CT in place of the more time-consuming transmission scan for attenuation correction. The ability to localize pathologic findings and to differentiate physiologic and pathologic tracer uptake[24,25] is also beneficial. Combined PET/MR machines have been introduced recently, and their value in clinical application is currently under investigation.[26] However, several problems due to patient movement can occur in hybrid imaging. First, despite shorter acquisition times, motion artifacts can appear in morphologic imaging modality as well as in PET. On CT images, mushroom-shaped artifacts due to respiration movement can typically be observed at the border of the lung and the liver (**Fig. 3**). In general, these artifacts can appear in all locations with moving borders between tissues of different attenuation properties.[27]

Of course, the above-mentioned artifacts in PET imaging will also appear in PET/CT and PET/MR imaging. However, there are additional motion artifacts that can solely be found in hybrid imaging (**Table 1**). As PET/CT is the standard in hybrid imaging, artifacts occurring in this modality are discussed, although most of the discussion can be extended to PET/MR imaging as well (**Fig. 4**).

The origin of motion artifacts in PET/CT is based on the difference in time resolution of the 2 imaging modalities. PET acquisition takes several minutes and consequently represents an averaged image over this time interval, whereas CT is acquired within several seconds and is therefore a snapshot of one motion state of the patient. Respiratory motion can lead to severe misalignment of PET and CT images (**Fig. 5**). These artifacts can be avoided or at least reduced using an optimal PET/CT acquisition protocol.[28] In the worst case, misalignment of PET and CT may lead to the assignment of PET findings to a wrong and healthy organ. Although these situations are rare, they are most likely to occur at the border between the liver and the lung and may lead to wrong diagnosis.[29] Bowel motion is another potential source of misdiagnosis; when focal PET uptake of a lymph node is projected to the bowel wall and hence classified wrongly as bowel uptake. Of course, misalignment of PET and CT has been reported in lung imaging since the introduction of hybrid scanners.[30] Cohade and colleagues[31] found in a study of 244 patients that a mean difference of 7.6 mm between the center of a lesion in PET and CT could be observed with an even more pronounced effect (10.2 mm) in the lower lobes of the lung (6.7 mm in the upper parts of the lung). Although misalignment in the lung does not frequently influence clinical diagnosis (as lung lesions normally can be aligned visually by the observer), it might change the quantification of PET data.

In hybrid imaging, anatomic image information is used for correction of PET data for photon attenuation and scatter effects.[10] While this is performed routinely in PET/CT, methods for attenuation correction using MR imaging in PET/MR are currently under investigation.[32,33] Thus, misalignment of morphologic imaging and PET data can lead to errors in correction of PET data and hence to wrong quantitative values in PET images. However, this problem can only be observed when different attenuation values appear in the area of misalignment, which is typically in the lung. Average attenuation values of the lung range from 0.005 to 0.05 cm^{-1}, whereas linear attenuation coefficients of soft tissue range between 0.09 and 0.11 cm^{-1}.[33] If, for example, attenuation values of lung tissue are assigned incorrectly to a PET-positive lung lesion, the attenuation coefficient and hence the resulting values of the attenuation-corrected PET images are underestimated (**Fig. 6**). The effect of such a false quantification was reported in Ref.[34] for a patient with an adenocarcinoma of the esophagogastric junction (AEG) underestimating the standardized uptake value (SUV) in the follow-up scan by 56% due to attenuation correction errors. Owing

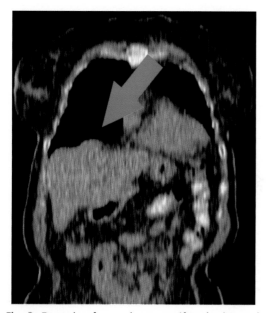

Fig. 3. Example of a mushroom artifact (*red arrow*) caused by movement of the liver dome during CT acquisition.

Table 1 Overview of motion artifacts		
Smearing of the lesion	Stand-alone PET and hybrid imaging	Detectability of small lesions is shortened due to reduced signal-to-noise ratio caused by smearing of the lesion Smearing of the lesions leads to false-large lesion volume and false-low tracer uptake in quantitative analysis
Misalignment of PET and morphologic imaging	Hybrid imaging	False assignment of pathologic PET uptake
	Hybrid imaging using CT or MRI for correction of PET data	Errors in quantification of tracer uptake when wrong attenuation coefficients are assigned to the lesion because of misalignment

to respiration and/or motion of the esophagus, the AEG was incorrectly assigned to lung tissue, which resulted in an undercorrection for attenuation. The baseline scan did not show any misalignment and PET uptake values were correct.

Cardiac Imaging

Cardiac PET is performed to diagnose several clinical conditions including myocardial ischemia or myocardial viability. Perfusion imaging under rest and stress conditions is performed using various tracers such as ^{82}Rb, ^{15}O-water, or ^{13}N-ammonia, whereas myocardial viability is derived from FDG images. In addition to the delineation of static tracer distribution as performed in conventional nuclear scintigraphy, PET data can be acquired dynamically. The latter approach allows, by using kinetic models, absolute measures of myocardial blood flow or myocardial metabolism.

As in oncological imaging, movement of the target structure itself, that is, the heart, leads to activity smearing. Thus, a static image always represents a mixture of information stemming from perfusion and wall motion. In addition, respiratory motion leads to a moderate blur along the body axis. Only limited implementations of respiratory cardiac triggering are[35] available, whereas ECG-gated acquisitions are performed routinely separating effectively cardiac motion and tracer uptake. Furthermore, the assessment of global and regional contractibility yields clinically useful and highly predictive parameters. However, this comes at the price that instead of 1 image 8 or even 16 frames need to be generated, thus reducing the signal-to-noise ratio of the individual frames. One potential solution is the concept of

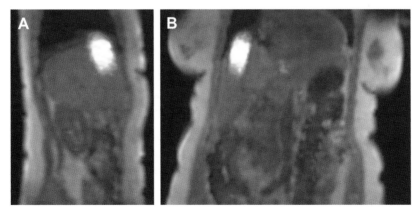

Fig. 4. Sagittal (A) and coronal (B) image of a fused PET/MR image of liver metastasis. Data was acquired on an integrated PET/MR system. However, MR and PET data were not acquired simultaneously, leading to typical artifacts due to respiratory movement: PET signal of the lesion is smeared. In addition, misalignment of the liver dome can be seen, especially in the sagittal orientation.

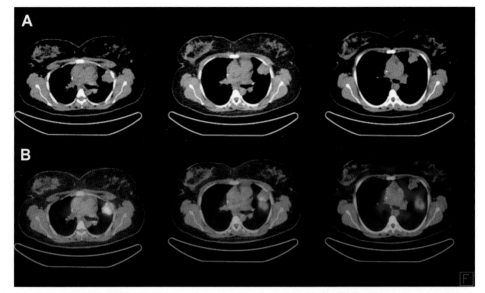

Fig. 5. CT (*A*) and fused PET/CT (*B*) of a lung metastasis of breast cancer. PET data was acquired without any motion compensation, whereas CT was acquired in 3 different breathing states (from left to right: expiration, mid-inspiration, inspiration). Obviously, only PET and CT data acquired in expiration can be coregistrated with less spatial mismatch, whereas there is significant misalignment in the other images.

"motion-frozen" data, which combines the gated images using nonrigid registration techniques to create one final, diastolic data set with increased spatial resolution and superior image quality compared to the gated[36] series.

Finally, misalignment of PET and anatomic data can induce artifacts because the latter is used for attenuation correction of the heart[37] and extensive underestimation of tracer uptake can arise especially in the free walls (**Fig. 7**).

Besides perfusion studies, imaging of vulnerable coronary plaques and vascular inflammation are becoming potential targets in PET imaging.[38] Most cases of myocardial infarction and sudden heart death are caused by a rupture of an atherosclerotic plaque. Thus early stratification is an important goal. However, calcification, size, or composition of the plaques or even the amount of luminal obstruction is not recognized to be a unique predictive factor for the risk of plaque rupture. Different PET tracers are under investigation for their diagnostic potential in plaque imaging and they target processes such as inflammation or neo-angiogenesis.[39] However, both coronary arteries and plaques, which are very small structures—at least from the perspective of PET imaging with a spatial resolution of about 6 mm, are constantly moving. It was shown that the localization of coronary arteries can change up to 23 mm during a heart cycle.[40] In a study by Delso and colleagues[41]

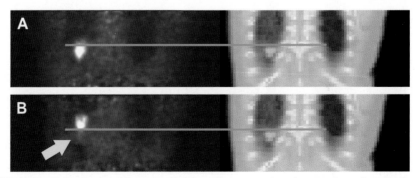

Fig. 6. FDG-PET image in inspiration (*A*) and expiration (*B*) compared to the corresponding CT slice (acquired in inspiration only). Using CT for attenuation correction of expiration PET data (*B*) resulted in an underestimation of activity uptake of the lesion of 16.2%. In addition, the erroneously high attenuation correction of background uptake in the lesion visible on CT can induce incorrectly high PET uptake values (*yellow arrow*).

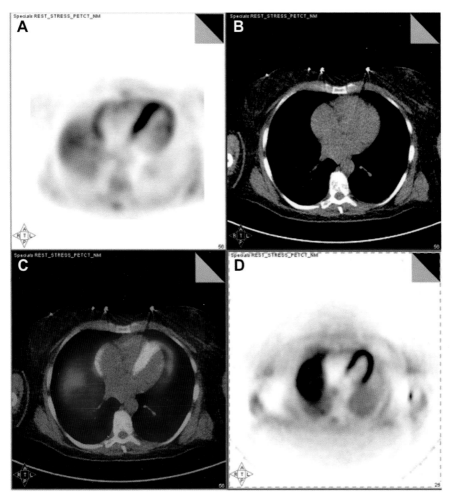

Fig. 7. Attenuation-corrected PET (*A*) and corresponding CT (*B*) of a cardiac study. The reduced tracer uptake in the lateral wall indicates a clear myocardial defect. However, in the fused image (*C*) misalignment probably due to respiratory movement is clearly visible, and if the non–attenuation-corrected image (*D*) is considered, a homogeneous tracer distribution over the wall of the left ventricle is visible. Therefore, the defect found in the attenuation-corrected image is induced by wrong attenuation correction arising from a motion artifact.

radioactive spheres of 1 mm size were placed to pig hearts in a surgical procedure followed by in vivo PET imaging including variable background activity by injection of ^{13}N-ammonia. The spheres were found to move up to 6.8 mm because of respiratory movement and up to 7.0 mm due to the heart beat. Depending on the variable signal-to-background activity due to the decaying ^{13}N-ammonia, some spheres were not visible as a consequence of motion blur. In contrast, post mortem, all spheres were visible as it was the case when combined cardiac and respiratory gating was used.[41]

The advantages of dynamic PET images have been mentioned before, and gross patient motion is an obvious obstacle for the quantification of these studies. Unfortunately, only limited information is available.[42,43] However, simultaneous PET/MR

systems could offer a significant improvement because patient movement could be monitored noninvasively by means of MR imaging, as initial studies[44] show.

SUMMARY

Patient movement is one of the most important limiting factors in qualitative as well as quantitative image analysis of PET. In PET images, motion blur leads to an underestimation of the tracer activity in the structures and an overestimation of the structure volume. Small structures may not be resolved against the background at all. In hybrid imaging, motion can occur between morphologic and functional imaging. This motion may result in the wrong localization of pathologic findings or, if anatomic imaging data are used for attenuation correction, in hampered quantification of PET data.

REFERENCES

1. Hicks RJ. Beyond FDG: novel PET tracers for cancer imaging. Cancer Imaging 2004;4:22–4.
2. Haubner R. PET radiopharmaceuticals in radiation treatment planning - synthesis and biological characteristics. Radiother Oncol 2010;96:280–7.
3. Jakoby BW, Bercier Y, Watson CC, et al. Performance characteristics of a new LSO PET/CT scanner with extended axial field-of-view and PSF reconstruction. IEEE Trans Nucl Sci 2009;56:633–9.
4. Jakoby BW, Bercier Y, Conti M, et al. Physical and clinical performance of the mCT time-of-flight PET/CT scanner. Phys Med Biol 2011;56:2375–89.
5. Surti S, Scheuermann J, El Fakhri G, et al. Impact of time-of-flight PET on whole-body oncologic studies: a human observer lesion detection and localization study. J Nucl Med 2011;52:712–9.
6. Townsend DW, Beyer T, Blodgett TM. PET/CT scanners: a hardware approach to image fusion. Semin Nucl Med 2003;33:193–204.
7. Nakamoto Y, Chin BB, Cohade C, et al. PET/CT: artifacts caused by bowel motion. Nucl Med Commun 2004;25:221–5.
8. Truong MT, Erasmus JJ, Munden RF, et al. Focal FDG uptake in mediastinal brown fat mimicking malignancy: a potential pitfall resolved on PET/CT. AJR Am J Roentgenol 2004;183:1127–32.
9. Hong TS, Shammas A, Charron M, et al. Brown adipose tissue 18F-FDG uptake in pediatric PET/CT imaging. Pediatr Radiol 2011;41:759–68.
10. Kinahan PE, Townsend DW, Beyer T, et al. Attenuation correction for a combined 3D PET/CT scanner. Med Phys 1998;25:2046–53.
11. Delso G, Ziegler S. PET/MRI system design. Eur J Nucl Med Mol Imaging 2009;36(Suppl 1):S86–92.
12. Brandner ED, Wu A, Chen H, et al. Abdominal organ motion measured using 4D CT. Int J Radiat Oncol Biol Phys 2006;65:554–60.
13. Suramo I, Paivansalo M, Myllyla V. Cranio-caudal movements of the liver, pancreas and kidneys in respiration. Acta Radiol Diagn (Stockh) 1984;25:129–31.
14. Bundschuh RA, Martinez-Moller A, Essler M, et al. Local motion correction for lung tumours in PET/CT-first results. Eur J Nucl Med Mol Imaging 2008;35:1981–8.
15. Plathow C, Ley S, Fink C, et al. Analysis of inthrathoracic tumor mobility during whole breathing cycle by dynamic MRI. Int J Radiat Oncol Biol Phys 2004;59:952–9.
16. Nehmeh SA, Erdi YE, Ling CC, et al. Effect of respiratory gating on reducing lung motion artifacts in PET imaging of lung cancer. Med Phys 2002;29:366–71.
17. Ott K, Weber WA, Lordick F, et al. Metabolic imaging predicts response, survival, and recurrence in adenocarcinomas of the esophagogastric junction. J Clin Oncol 2006;24:4692–8.
18. Weber WA, Wieder H. Monitoring chemotherapy and radiotherapy of solid tumors. Eur J Nucl Med Mol Imaging 2006;33(Suppl 1):27–37.
19. De Ruysscher D, Kirsch CM. PET scans in radiotherapy planning of lung cancer. Radiother Oncol 2010;96:335–8.
20. Astner ST, Dobrei-Ciuchendea M, Essler M, et al. Effect of 11C-methionine-positron emission tomography on gross tumor volume delineation in stereotactic radiotherapy of skull base meningiomas. Int J Radiat Oncol Biol Phys 2008;72:1161–7.
21. Eich HT, Muller RP, Engenhart-Cabillic R, et al. Involved-node radiotherapy in early-stage Hodgkin's lymphoma. Definition and guidelines of the German Hodgkin Study Group (GHSG). Strahlenther Onkol 2008;184:406–10.
22. Bundschuh RA, Andratschke N, Dinges J, et al. Respiratory gated [(18)F]FDG PET/CT for target volume delineation in stereotactic radiation treatment of liver metastases. Strahlenther Onkol 2012;188:592–8.
23. Astner ST, Bundschuh RA, Beer AJ, et al. Assessment of tumor volumes in skull base glomus tumors using Gluc-Lys[(18)F]-TOCA positron emission tomography. Int J Radiat Oncol Biol Phys 2009;73:1135–40.
24. Wahl RL. Why nearly all PET of abdominal and pelvic cancers will be performed as PET/CT. J Nucl Med 2004;45(Suppl 1):82S–95S.
25. Goerres GW, von Schulthess GK, Steinert HC. Why most PET of lung and head-and-neck cancer will be PET/CT. J Nucl Med 2004;45(Suppl 1):66S–71S.
26. Drzezga A, Souvatzoglou M, Eiber M, et al. First clinical experience with integrated whole-body PET/MR: comparison to PET/CT in patients with oncologic diagnoses. J Nucl Med 2012;53:845–55.
27. Chen GT, Kung JH, Beaudette KP. Artifacts in computed tomography scanning of moving objects. Semin Radiat Oncol 2004;14:19–26.
28. Beyer T, Antoch G, Muller S, et al. Acquisition protocol considerations for combined PET/CT imaging. J Nucl Med 2004;45(Suppl 1):25S–35S.
29. Sarikaya I, Yeung HW, Erdi Y, et al. Respiratory artefact causing malpositioning of liver dome lesion in right lower lung. Clin Nucl Med 2003;28:943–4.
30. Goerres GW, Kamel E, Seifert B, et al. Accuracy of image coregistration of pulmonary lesions in patients with non-small cell lung cancer using an integrated PET/CT system. J Nucl Med 2002;43:1469–75.

31. Cohade C, Osman M, Marshall LN, et al. PET-CT: accuracy of PET and CT spatial registration of lung lesions. Eur J Nucl Med Mol Imaging 2003;30:721–6.

32. Zaidi H. Is MR-guided attenuation correction a viable option for dual-modality PET/MR imaging? Radiology 2007;244:639–42.

33. Martinez-Moller A, Souvatzoglou M, Delso G, et al. Tissue classification as a potential approach for attenuation correction in whole-body PET/MRI: evaluation with PET/CT data. J Nucl Med 2009;50:520–6.

34. Bundschuh RA, Martinez-Moller A, Ziegler SI, et al. Misalignment in PET/CT: relevance for SUV and therapy management. Nuklearmedizin 2008;47:N14–5.

35. Martinez-Moller A, Zikic D, Botnar RM, et al. Dual cardiac-respiratory gated PET: implementation and results from a feasibility study. Eur J Nucl Med Mol Imaging 2007;34:1447–54.

36. Le Meunier L, Slomka PJ, Dey D, et al. Motion frozen (18)F-FDG cardiac PET. J Nucl Cardiol 2011;18:259–66.

37. Martinez-Möller A, Souvatzoglou M, Navab N, et al. Artifacts from misaligned CT in cardiac perfusion PET/CT studies: frequency, effects, and potential solutions. J Nucl Med 2007;48:188–93.

38. Schwaiger M, Ziegler SI, Nekolla SG. PET/CT challenge for the non-invasive diagnosis of coronary artery disease. Eur J Radiol 2010;73:494–503.

39. Saraste A, Nekolla SG, Schwaiger M. Cardiovascular molecular imaging: an overview. Cardiovasc Res 2009;83:643–52.

40. Wang Y, Vidan E, Bergman GW. Cardiac motion of coronary arteries: variability in the rest period and implications for coronary MR angiography. Radiology 1999;213:751–8.

41. Delso G, Martinez-Moller A, Bundschuh RA, et al. Preliminary study of the detectability of coronary plaque with PET. Phys Med Biol 2011;56:2145–60.

42. Woo J, Tamarappoo B, Dey D, et al. Automatic 3D registration of dynamic stress and rest (82)Rb and flurpiridaz F 18 myocardial perfusion PET data for patient motion detection and correction. Med Phys 2011;38:6313–26.

43. Koshino K, Watabe H, Enmi J, et al. Effects of patient movement on measurements of myocardial blood flow and viability in resting (1)(5)O-water PET studies. J Nucl Cardiol 2012;19:524–33.

44. Chun SY, Reese TG, Ouyang J, et al. MRI-based nonrigid motion correction in simultaneous PET/MRI. J Nucl Med 2012;53:1284–91.

Motion-Tracking Hardware and Advanced Applications in PET and PET/CT

V. Bettinardi, MSc[a,b,*], E. De Bernardi, PhD[a,c,d],
L. Presotto, MSc[a,e], M.C. Gilardi, MSc[a,b,c,d]

KEYWORDS

- Gating technology • Hybrid PET/computed tomography • Motion monitoring and tracking devices

KEY POINTS

- Respiratory and cardiac motions represent important sources of image degradation in both PET and computed tomography (CT) studies that need to be taken into account and compensated.
- An advanced strategy to account and compensate for respiratory and cardiac motion is to acquire PET and CT data in gating mode.
- Motion monitoring and tracking devices used in PET and CT gating studies are important tools for performing respiratory and cardiac gating studies.

INTRODUCTION

The respiratory and cardiac motions of patients represent important sources of degradation for both image quality and quantitative accuracy of oncologic and cardiac PET studies.[1–10] Motion during data acquisition induces a spread of the true radioactivity distribution, which results in tracer uptake underestimation and volume overestimation for the organ or lesion of interest.[3,4] Furthermore, in the case of hybrid PET/computed tomography (CT) studies, respiratory and cardiac motions are also responsible for temporal/spatial mismatches between PET and CT data, owing to the different acquisition times. In fact, multislice CT scanners allow whole-body studies to be performed in a few seconds (eg,10–30 seconds) thus freezing, in the CT images, the anatomy of the patient at a specific moment of the respiratory cycle. Conversely, whole-body PET studies require a longer scan time (2–3 minutes for bed position, 15–20 minutes for the whole body), which results in PET images showing a lesion as a blurred radioactivity distribution averaged over several breathing cycles (eg, 30–45). Because in hybrid PET/CT systems the CT images are used for the attenuation correction of the PET data, such incoherencies between CT and PET can produce artifacts on the reconstructed PET images.[5–8] It is worth noting that important technological innovations aimed at improving the accuracy of PET images, such as spatial resolution and signal-to-noise ratio, can be partially if not completely nullified by such motion effects.

To account and compensate for respiratory or cardiac motion, PET and CT data can be acquired in gating mode (also named 4-dimensional [4D] acquisition mode).[9,10] The idea behind gating is

[a] Department of Nuclear Medicine, Ospedale San Raffaele, via Olgettina 60, 20132 Segrate, Milano, Italy; [b] IBFM-CNR, Institute for Molecular Bioimaging and Physiology, via Fratelli Cervi 93, 20132 Segrate, Milano, Italy; [c] Department of Health Sciences University of Milano-Bicocca, via Cadore 48, 20090 Monza, Monza e Brianza, Italy; [d] Tecnomed Foundation, University of Milano-Bicocca, via Pergolesi 33, 20090 Monza, Monza Brianza, Italy; [e] Department of Physics G. Occhialini, University of Milano Bicocca, Piazza della Scienza 3, 20126 Milano, Italy
* Corresponding author.
E-mail address: bettinardi.valentino@hsr.it

PET Clin 8 (2013) 11–28
http://dx.doi.org/10.1016/j.cpet.2012.09.008
1556-8598/13/$ – see front matter © 2013 Elsevier Inc. All rights reserved.

to synchronize the acquisition of the data to a description of the organ/lesion movement, by "observing," in a noninvasive way, the patient from outside the body. Motion-tracking systems (MTSs) are therefore required to measure representative external signals assessing the organ/lesion motion during the whole data-acquisition process.

In 4D oncologic studies, the respiratory movement must be considered; in 4D cardiac studies both respiratory and cardiac movements must be taken into account.

In diagnostic clinical oncology or follow-up studies, gating may be used to obtain motion-free PET and CT images as well as truly spatially coregistered PET and CT data, thus improving both image quality and quantitative accuracy.[9,10]

Gating is also very important in PET and PET/CT studies for radiation therapy (RT) applications, to acquire a full knowledge of tumor and surrounding organ motion during the whole respiratory cycle. This information can be very useful in improving the definition of target volume and in personalizing the treatment plan, to increase the dose to the tumor and to reduce that to surrounding healthy tissues and organs at risk.[11–14]

Gating may be implemented in prospective or retrospective mode. In prospective gating, multiple fixed partitions covering the whole breathing/cardiac cycle or a single specific partition (eg, end of the expiration, end of the diastolic phase) are set before starting data acquisition. Data acquisition is then triggered by the acquired signal. Nowadays prospective gating with a single partition is the acquisition technique most commonly used to obtain motion-free images representative of a specific moment of the physiologic process. Conversely, in retrospective gating, data are collected during the whole breathing/cardiac cycle and only subsequently sorted into the established number of partitions, according to the recorded signal.

The choice and detection of the signal representative of the physiologic effect under consideration (respiration, cardiac beat) is a very important step in the gating technique. In cardiac studies the electrical activity of the heart represents a natural signal to be used for gating. By contrast, for breathing there is a no well-codified physical effect that can be easily detected from outside the patient. Therefore, to assess the breathing-cycle movements in PET and PET/CT respiratory gating, several MTSs have been designed and evaluated. Differences between MTSs essentially relate to the kind of physiologic signal monitored (eg, air flux, lung volume, abdominal displacement) and the signal-processing method.

The recorded signal can in fact be processed by phase or amplitude. In phase-based gating, each cycle is divided into a defined number of partitions (phases) by considering only the temporal information associated to the signal, independently from its amplitude. This type of data processing has been demonstrated to work well for patients with a regular respiratory cycle, but results in motion artifacts in patients with irregular patterns.[15,16] By contrast, amplitude-based gating techniques divide the total respiration amplitude into different gates (bins) independently of the time information associated with the signal. It has been shown that amplitude-gating techniques are more robust than phase-gating techniques, thus allowing for a better suppression of motion artifacts.[15,16] As an alternative to gating, in cases of respiratory motion, breath-hold (BH) methods have been recently proposed, whereby the patient is asked to hold his or her breath with the aim of achieving tumor immobilization: (1) at a specific moment of the breathing cycle (end inspiration, end expiration, and so forth) and (2) for a predefined time duration (eg, 10 seconds, 20 seconds, as long as possible).[17,18]

Whatever the acquisition and processing techniques used to perform a respiratory or cardiac PET or CT gating study, a fundamental component in performing such protocols is represented by the MTS, which is needed to synchronize the acquisition of the data (PET events or CT images) with the physiologic signal representing the patient's respiration or the patient's heart beating. The monitoring and tracking system in fact represents the interface between the acquisition system, PET or CT, and the patient.

The aim of this review is to describe and compare MTSs for 4D-PET and 4D-PET/CT. Commercial and research devices specifically proposed for monitoring and tracking respiratory/cardiac motion in PET and PET/CT applications, as well as systems designed to assess and monitor patient setup and patient movement in RT, but showing the potential to be also useful for PET and PET/CT studies, are taken into consideration. In the last section, advanced applications of the gating technique and the technological developments necessary to fully exploit its potential are discussed.

RESPIRATORY MONITORING AND TRACKING SYSTEMS FOR 4D-PET AND 4D-PET/CT

Breathing is an active process requiring the contraction of skeletal muscles. The muscles mainly involved in respiration are the external intercostal muscles and the diaphragm. During inspiration such muscles contract, inducing an elevation of ribs and sternum and a drawdown of the diaphragm, corresponding respectively to a front-to-back and vertical increase of the dimension of the thoracic cavity. The consequent reduction of the air pressure in the lungs determines the entry of the outside air. During expiration muscles relax and the diaphragm, ribs, and sternum return to the rest position, thus restoring the thoracic cavity to the preinspiratory volume. The consequent increase in air pressure in the lungs forces air expulsion.

The design of a respiratory MTS (RMTS) can rely on monitoring the physiologic signal associated with the internal changes of the lung volume or to the external changes in the shape of the thoracic or abdominal region.[19,20] Whereas the first solution is directly associated with the physiologic process of respiration, the second detects only a surrogate of the true respiratory signal. A critical issue of each RMTS is the assumption that the detected signal correlates well with the true motion of the organ and tumor under investigation,[21–23] therefore the choice of the signal to be monitored must be carefully considered.

Other aspects that must be taken into account in the design of an RMTS are: (1) invasiveness, (2) patient comfort, (3) adaptability, and (4) ease of setting and handling for both the patient and the technicians.[24,25] Furthermore, the system should be highly reliable (hardware and software), accurate, and reproducible in all the different possible working conditions. In particular, the sensor used to monitor and track the target signal should (1) respond quickly to variations of the signal, (2) not introduce drifts in the signal baseline, (3) have a high signal-to-noise ratio, and (4) not produce artifacts on the acquired images.[24,25]

SPIROMETER

The spirometer is a device that measures volume and the rate of air flow inspired and expired by the lungs, and so theoretically is the ideal RMTS.[24–27] The more general configuration of a spirometer consists of a reservoir for air collection connected by means of a tube to a mouthpiece through which the patient is asked to breathe, along with a nasal clip used to avoid nasal breathing. The tube is generally equipped with a differential pressure sensor that converts the air flow into a pressure signal, which is transformed into an analog electric signal and finally digitized.[26]

The use of the spirometer as RMTS is based on the assumption that a direct correlation exists between lung volume, lung motion, and tumor position. This assumption has been verified in several articles by using fluoroscopy, CT, or other imaging techniques, mainly in oncologic lung studies.[28–30] However, a good correlation has also been shown for pancreas, liver, and breast.[30–32] Another advantage of the spirometer is the good reproducibility of the breathing signal in different breathing sessions.[31,33] For these reasons the spirometer has been used in several RT applications to optimize the treatment by reducing organ and tumor motion. In particular, it has been used in BH protocols to achieve tumor immobilization and reproducibility of the tumor position. However, the spirometer also has some drawbacks. The first of these is signal baseline drift, which particularly affects lengthy sessions and is due to different causes depending on the specific model of spirometer (eg, flow-sensitivity calibration error, imperfect zero-flow adjustment, nonlinear response to different flow rates).[26,34] The baseline drift, if not properly accounted for and compensated, results in a wrong estimate of the lung volume and consequently in a wrong estimate of the tumor position. The second drawback regards the relative "invasiveness" and discomfort of the spirometer, which forces the patient to breathe only with the mouth for a relatively long period of time. Furthermore, the setup of a spirometer requires a longer time for patient preparation relative to other systems, not least because the patient should be allowed to become used to this type of breathing before starting the study session.

At present, to the authors' knowledge, no commercial devices based on a spirometer are interfaced with any PET or PET/CT system. The use of the spirometer as an RMTS for PET gating has been described only in 2 studies, with controversial results. Martinez-Möller and colleagues[35] evaluated the spirometer and other devices as potential sensors for respiratory gating in emission tomography. In their experience the spirometer was discarded after measurement with volunteers because of its lower reliability. Noponen and colleagues,[36] by contrast, used a spirometer for respiratory gating in cardiac PET and magnetic resonance imaging, and reported a positive experience, concluding that it could be used to accurately follow respiratory motion.

MONODIMENSIONAL RESPIRATORY MONITORING AND TRACKING SYSTEMS: COMMERCIAL DEVICES

Commercial RMTSs are based on the detection of a surrogate of the breathing signal to make the RMTS easy to use and well tolerated by the patient. Most of the commercial devices were originally developed for RT systems and only recently have been interfaced with PET and PET/CT systems.[19,20]

Real-Time Position Management System

The real-time position management system (RPM; Varian Medical Systems, Palo Alto, CA, USA) is the most used, evaluated, and compared RMTS for both clinical and research applications.[19,20,37–43] RPM is a noninvasive, optoelectronic system based on a charge-coupled device (CCD) sensitive to infrared (IR) and visible light, whose lenses are surrounded by a matrix of infrared light-emitting diodes (LEDs). The camera, firmly attached to the patient table, illuminates a marker block, which is usually positioned on the patient's abdomen near the point of maximum excursion. On the surface of the marker block, facing the video camera, there are 2 passive reflective markers (circular dots of 5 mm in diameter, with 3 cm distance between the 2 dots). The upper marker is used to track the respiratory motion while the lower one is used to calibrate the system. When the patient breathes, the block follows the motion of the abdomen, and the system, by the simultaneous tracking of the light reflected by the 2 markers, detects the vertical component of the motion and maintains the calibration. In this way a monodimensional signal surrogate of the patient's respiratory signal is generated (**Fig. 1**). The RPM sampling frequency is 25–30 Hz. The recorded signal is processed and presented (in real time) as a waveform on the display of a personal computer. Recently, a new version of RPM that uses 6 passive markers has been made commercially available allowing for finer tracking (in 3 dimensions) of the patient's breathing. The RPM system can perform both prospectively or retrospectively, in phase or amplitude gating mode, depending on the third-party imaging system's characteristics (hardware and software). When set for prospective gating, RPM establishes synchronization by controlling the image-acquisition process. In particular, it outputs a trigger pulse whenever the phase or amplitude of the respiration signal crosses a user-specified level. The imaging device responds to the trigger

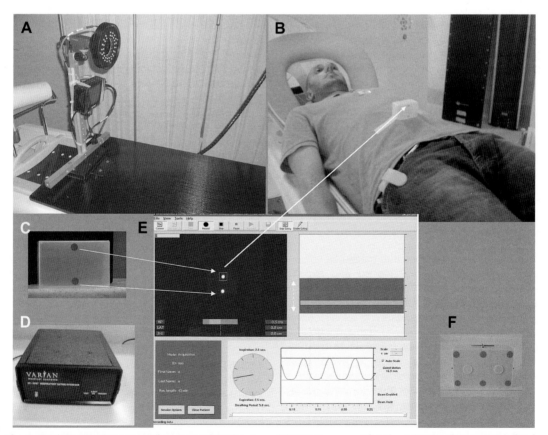

Fig. 1. Real-time positioning management (RPM) system. (*A*) CCD Camera with infrared LEDs. The camera is firmly attached to the patient's bed. (*B*) Subject in position on the scanner bed. Note the RPM box positioned in the region of his abdomen. (*C*) RPM plastic marker box (2-marker version). (*D*) Varian interface box. (*E*) Typical RPM interface. (*F*) RPM box (6-marker version).

and starts or stops the image acquisition. When set for retrospective gating, RPM and the imaging device exchange pulses that are recorded by either or both systems as synchronization tags. Once image acquisition is finished, the synchronization tags are used to correlate the acquired images/data with the phase or amplitude of the breathing signal recorded by RPM. In case of phase-mode analysis, values originally established in real time during acquisition can be recomputed at the end of the study, thus allowing a sorting of data better correlated with the respiratory phases. In general, all the information recorded by RPM during a study, as well as the input-output synchronization signals, are stored in a file, which may be edited and used for postprocessing of data.

The correlation between the external surrogate signal recorded by RPM and the internal tumor motion was evaluated by Chi and colleagues[44] and Beddar and colleagues[23] for lung and liver tumors, respectively. Specifically, Chi and colleagues[44] studied the relation between external surface motion and internal tumor motion by using cine images acquired with a 4D-CT protocol. The study showed that respiratory waveforms measured at different surface locations during the same respiratory cycle often varied and had significant phase shifts. The best correlation (smallest phase shift) was found between the abdominal motion and the superior-inferior tumor motion. This result supports the importance of placing the RPM block in the abdominal region as well as that of reproducing the same position of the block on the patient when the RPM system is used for RT. A similar study by Beddar and colleagues[23] investigated the correlation between the motion of an external marker and internal fiducials implanted in the liver for patients undergoing respiratory 4D-CT. The investigators found a good correlation between internal fiducial motion, imaged by 4D-CT, and external marker motion, with the best result at the end of the respiratory cycle.

ANZAI (AZ-733V) System

Another popular commercial RMTS is the Anzai (AZ-733V) system (Anzai Medical, Tokyo, Japan).[19,39,40] A pressure signal measured by a load cell inserted into a belt fastened around the patient's chest/abdomen is considered as a surrogate of the respiratory signal. When the patient breathes, the expansion of the thorax changes the tension of the belt, which in turn induces a change of pressure in the load cell. The sampling frequency of AZ-733V is 40 Hz. The system is delivered with 2 load cells with different sensitivities and with 4 belts of different

length. The AZ-7333V needs to be calibrated before each use. The calibration is performed using a load-cell calibrator which, once positioned on the load cell, produces a reference signal that can be adjusted on the rear side of the sensor port, which in turn is connected to a wave deck. The wave deck performs the analog-to-digital conversion of the signal and generates the trigger for the imaging system. It is connected to a computer where the information detected by the pressure sensor is displayed as the patient's respiratory curve (**Fig. 2**). As for the RPM, once interfaced with an imaging system (PET, CT), AZ-733V can perform either prospectively or retrospectively, in phase or amplitude gating mode, depending on the third-party imaging system's characteristics (hardware and software). All the information recorded by AZ-733V during a study as well as the input-output synchronization signals are stored in a file, which may be edited and used for postprocessing of data.

Even if both RPM and AZ-733V can be interfaced with most imaging and RT systems, sometimes, owing to technological incompatibilities, the same device cannot be used over the entire chain of diagnostic/simulation and treatment sessions. In this regard Li and colleagues,[39] and later Otani and colleagues,[40] evaluated the level of correlation between the surrogate respiratory signals generated by the two systems, to assess the possibility of using one device in the diagnostic/simulation session and the other in the treatment sessions. Both studies revealed a strong correlation between the two signals (99%). Li and colleagues[39] concluded that 4D-CT data sets acquired with RPM could be used to design gated treatments to be performed with AZ-733V. Otani and colleagues,[40] however, observed that during irregular breathing periods tags generated in phase mode by the two systems were different, thus inducing differences in centroid position of tumor and estimation of tumor shape.

Bellows System

The respiratory bellows system (RBS; Medspira, Minneapolis, MN, USA) is a device constituted by a bellows attached to a belt.[45–47] The belt is fastened around the patient with the bellows positioned on the chest/abdomen. A breathing signal is generated as result of the expansion and contraction of the chest/abdomen during inspiration and expiration. In particular, a variation in the length of the bellows during patient's breathing causes a change in the air pressure within the tube, which is measured by a pressure-sensitive transducer. The pressure signal is therefore the surrogate of

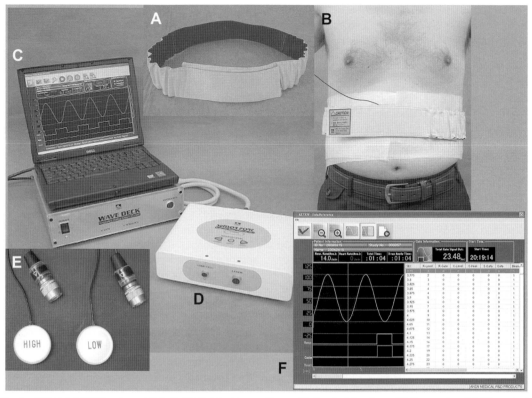

Fig. 2. ANZAI AZ-733V system. (*A*) Belt. (*B*) Subject in position with the belt in place. (*C*) Computer. (*D*) Wave deck. (*E*) Load sensors. (*F*) AZ-733V interface.

the respiratory signal, which is digitalized, and transmitted to the imaging system (eg, PET, CT) and to a Mayo Clinic respiratory feedback system (MCRFS; Mayo Clinic, Rochester, MN, USA). The MCRFS comprises monitors displaying LEDs, which give continuous real-time feedback on the respiratory function to both operator and patient (**Fig. 3**). The operator must define a reference position (central LED) by pressing a reference button at the desired point of the respiratory cycle. In case of free-breathing sessions the reference position must correspond to the midpoint between maximum inhalation and maximum exhalation. The patient is then instructed to light up the same number of LEDs at full inspiration as at full expiration, relative to the central LED. In case of an uneven number of lights, which usually indicates an uncomfortable breathing pattern for the patient, the operator can adjust the reference position to determine a new, more comfortable breathing condition. For BH sessions, the reference position must correspond to the desired BH level. The patient is then instructed to stop breathing only when the central LED is illuminated. Illumination of LEDs above or below the middle LED indicates greater or lesser degrees of inspiration, respectively. Before each study the bellows

must be reset by pushing a button on the base unit, which equalizes the air pressure in the tube. As for RPM and AZ-733V, the bellows system can perform either prospectively or retrospectively in phase or amplitude gating mode, depending on the third-party imaging system's characteristics.

Originally the bellows system was developed and validated for intermittent-mode CT fluoroscopy–guided biopsy by Carlson and colleagues.[45] In this study, the system showed: (1) high sensitivity, as body wall motions up to a nominal level of 1 mm were consistently detected; (2) high reliability, as small coefficient of variations (1.9%, 1.4%, 0.7%, 0.8%, and 0.7%) were found for multiple displacements levels (3.6, 6.0, 10, 15, and 20 mm); (3) ease of setup and use for both physicians and patients; and (4) high correlation between BH levels and internal target location ($r^2 = 0.84–0.94$).

MONODIMENSIONAL RESPIRATORY MONITORING AND TRACKING SYSTEMS: RESEARCH DEVICES

Until recently, most of the commercial RMTSs interfaced with hybrid PET/CT scanners allowed only a phase-based gating of PET/CT data. This

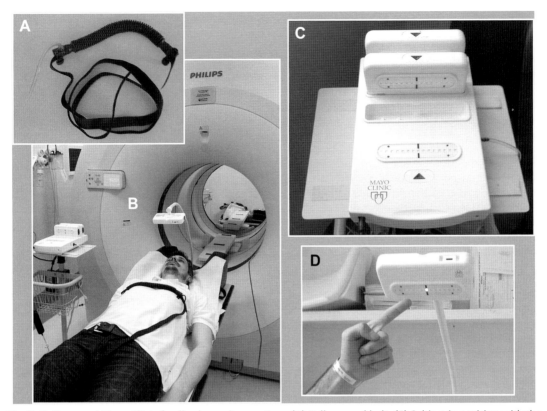

Fig. 3. Bellows and Mayo Clinic feedback monitors system. (*A*) Bellows and belt. (*B*) Subject in position with the bellows and the Mayo Clinic feedback monitors in place. (*C*) Mayo Clinic feedback base monitor units. (*D*) Single monitor with central LED turned on.

sorting technique has been demonstrated to be accurate in case of regular breathing patterns, but suboptimal in presence of breathing irregularities.[15,16] For this reason, the development of new and more flexible RMTSs able to perform also amplitude-based gating has been a very active research area over the last few years.

In this regard, Chang and colleagues[48] proposed a device designed specifically to perform free-breathing amplitude gating (FBAG) in PET/CT diagnostic applications. The changes in the thoracic/abdominal circumference during breathing are measured through a respiratory belt transducer, which contains a piezoelectric element converting pressure into an electric signal. The ability of the device to correctly detect the respiratory waveform was demonstrated by comparing the signal and its Fourier transform with those simultaneously obtained with the AZ-7333V system on 10 volunteers (correlation coefficients 0.86 ± 0.08 and 0.94 ± 0.03, respectively). During the whole data-acquisition process, patients were allowed to breathe freely. By a graphic user interface the system allows display of the detected respiratory signal and injection of a 5-V transistor-transistor logic trigger signal

into the PET list stream whenever the signal amplitude crosses the established respiratory amplitude range. The acquisition stops when the total accumulated time in the selected amplitude range reaches a predetermined value. The PET list stream is then retrospectively filtered to select only the events falling within the amplitude range, and data rebinned with standard PET/CT scanner software.[48,49]

Another RMTS specifically developed for amplitude-based gating of PET/CT studies is the multidimensional respiratory tracking (MDRT) system, recently proposed by Nehmeh and colleagues.[50] With the MDRT system the investigators also implemented and evaluated a new acquisition protocol for motion-free PET data, namely smart gating, which allows data to be prospectively acquired only at an user-specified breathing amplitude, avoiding additional postprocessing. The MDRT system acquires 2-dimensional (2D) breathing-motion information using a commercial video camera, which tracks the movement of multiple landmarks positioned on the patient's abdomen. Images acquired by the video camera are recorded in real time, with an average frequency of 25 Hz. At the beginning of the study, the operator identifies each marker by placing a region of interest on the images. Markers are then tracked in real time as 2D spatial coordinates (x and y) on a frame-by-frame basis. The displacement of the markers along the y direction is the surrogate respiratory signal. The accuracy of MDRT in tracking the breathing signal was assessed (1) by comparing the period of an oscillating phantom with that measured with a photogate timer (errors <2%), and (2) by comparing the registered respiratory waveform with that detected by RPM on 10 patients (percent error in the peaks' position <10%). Amplitude gating is obtained by defining an amplitude threshold window. As long as the breathing signal is within the amplitude window, MDRT sends a trigger every 4 milliseconds to the PET scanner and acquires data accumulated into a unique amplitude-gated bin. When the breathing signal falls outside the amplitude window, MDRT stops sending the trigger and data acquisition is suspended until a new trigger arrives. The patient is instructed to perform a BH as long as possible at a specific amplitude. If the patient fails to hold the breath, he or she is allowed to breathe normally for few seconds before being guided again. The amplitude-based control of the BH is more robust than the standard BH protocol, whereby the patient is simply asked to hold the breath at a specific amplitude for a predefined period of time. Once the acquisition is terminated no further processing is needed, as during the acquisition only correct data have been recorded.

TOWARD MULTIDIMENSIONAL FULL MONITORING AND TRACKING OF PATIENT MOVEMENT

Monodimensional RMTSs assume that the position of lesions and internal organs during the image-acquisition period correlates with the amplitude of a single 1-dimensional signal taken as a surrogate description of the patient breathing. For PET and PET/CT gating this kind of modeling has been demonstrated to be sufficient in most cases; however, it might fail in presence of changes in the breathing pattern (eg, from abdominal to chest and vice versa) as well as in cases of patient movements other than breathing. In RT and stereotactic surgery applications, where a high accuracy in the assessment of the position of organs and lesions is required, multidimensional MTSs able to obtain a full 3-dimensional (3D) description of the patient movement have been introduced. These systems are generally based on optical technology using more than 1 video camera to track multiple markers positioned on the patient's skin or directly image

the surface of the patient's chest/abdomen. Multidimensional MTSs are able to generate a reconstruction of the patient's positioning in 3D space and, with an adequate temporal sampling, to monitor the patient's movements and respiratory pattern.[51,52] These systems may be considered as overdesigned for daily usage in diagnostic PET and gated PET/CT studies, but the introduction of some kind of simplified version may be desirable in PET and PET/CT, in particular when used for RT planning purposes. In the following, a brief description is provided of some of these multidimensional MTSs that may potentially lead to a more general management of patient motion in 4D-PET and 4D-PET/CT.

ExactTrac (ET; Brainlab, Feldkirchen, Germany) is an IR-based optical positioning system constituted by 2 IR video cameras mounted on the ceiling of the treatment room, tracking a set of 5 to 7 passive optical body markers positioned on the patient's thorax.[20,53–59] Once calibrated, ET assesses the position of each marker in 3D space with respect to the isocenter of the RT system with a sampling frequency of 20 to 30 Hz. In image-guided RT applications, ET is coupled with a set of radiographic kV x-ray devices in double-oblique projection to determine the position of internal anatomy relative to the isocenter. In particular, the radiographic kV device consists of 2 floor-mounted diagnostic kV x-ray tubes and 2 corresponding ceiling-mounted amorphous silicon x-ray imagers. In this configuration, the ET system is used for precise targeting with respect to the patient's bony anatomy as well as for patient positioning relative to internal movable soft tissues. Once in the treatment room, the ET continuously tracks the markers on the patient's skin to establish the correct patient position relative to the isocenter of the treatment system.[51] The patient setup is performed in the following steps: (1) automatic patient alignment by the optical system (along the 3 linear directions); and (2) acquisition of 2 orthogonal kV images and automatic matching with the reference digitally reconstructed radiograph images (calculated from the CT images acquired during the simulation/planning session) for the assessment of 6 setup correction parameters (3 translation and 3 rotations) able to compensate for internal misalignments. Because soft-tissue targets may not be well visualized on planar radiographs, implanted fiducials may be used.[52] Once the setup procedure is completed, ET allows the real-time monitoring of the patient's position with respect to that established for the treatment. Furthermore, the ET system allows tracking of the respiratory motion from the average movement of the surface body markers. In particular, the respiratory signal can be detected and tracked to control the RT beam in a gating procedure, allowing the beam to be ON only during the desired portion of the respiratory cycle. The same gating signal is used to control the "beam ON/OFF" of the x-ray imaging devices to allow x-ray tracking of implanted radiopaque markers during treatment.[52]

An assessment of the accuracy of ET and RPM in respiratory motion tracking was recently performed by Chang and colleagues.[41] Artificial motion patterns and true patient respiratory profiles were evaluated by comparing the motion trajectories acquired by the two gating systems against the references. Results show that both systems can reliably track respiratory motion: by considering a maximum motion amplitude of 28.0 mm, the average mean discrepancy respect to the reference was 1.5 and 1.9 mm for ET and 1.1 and 1.7 mm for RPM, for artificial and patient profiles, respectively.

GateCT (VisionRT, London, UK) is another optical monitoring and tracking system that is able to track the patient's movements in 3D and in real time. It acquires surface images (eg, a region of the patient's chest) that are used to verify patient setup as well as to monitor patient motion.[20,60–62]

The system is constituted by a 3D stereoscopic camera, which contains a projector that projects a pattern of light on the patient's chest/abdomen region, and by 2 CCD cameras that acquire the pattern (**Fig. 4**). Patient and respiratory motion are independently tracked. Therefore, once the reference surface has been acquired, the user must manually select a set of tracking points for detection of patient motion and a second set for detection of respiratory motion. In particular, the respiratory points should be chosen over a region where a clear breathing signal is expected, and stable points exhibiting minimal motion (eg, points over bony landmark) should be selected as motion points. The sampling frequency depends on the size of the detected area; for example, for a standard region of 20×20 mm^2, a sampling rate of 16 Hz is used. The temporal and spatial accuracy of GateCT in tracking the respiratory signal was assessed by Kauweloa and colleagues.[42] GateCT and RPM were compared on simulated breathing patterns (ideal/nonideal), and on real patient respiratory curves. GateCT revealed its consistency in temporal/phase tracking, but appeared less accurate than RPM in detecting the absolute abdominal position, in particular for low-amplitude breathing patterns. Vàsquez and

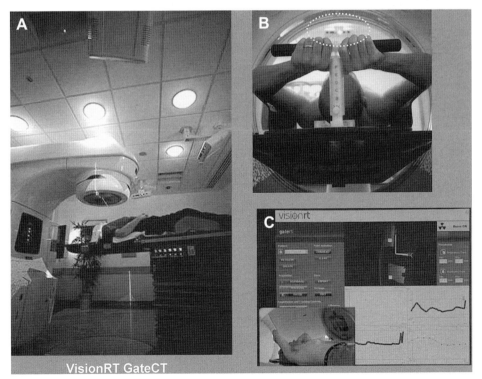

Fig. 4. GateCT system (VisionRT). (*A*) Simulation room with the GateCT system in place. (*B*) Patient in position for RT simulation. Note the GateCT system (*white elliptical dotted area*) monitoring the patient. (*C*) Typical GateCT interface.

colleagues[62] assessed instead the suitability of GateCT as RMTS for amplitude-based gating in 4D-CT and compared its performance with AZ-733V. In this study, both systems were able to generate 4D-CT images free of motion artifact, provided that a regular sampling and a correct setting of the sampling rate were imposed.

In recent years many multidimensional optical MTSs have been proposed in the literature, with the common aim of contemporaneously tracking different aspects of patient movement.[63–67]

One example of these multidimensional and multitasking optical tracking systems has been developed and evaluated by Lyatskaya and colleagues.[66] The system, specifically designed for RT applications, aims at a simultaneous and real-time monitoring of: (1) accuracy of patient's positioning with respect to RT system isocenter, (2) patient's posture (ie, body configuration with respect to the table), and (3) patient's breathing. The system consists of 2 IR video cameras (passive Polaris NDI model P4) mounted on the ceiling of the RT room, and of a set of passive reflective markers positioned on the patient's skin. Once calibrated, the system can track in real time (data collection frequency of 10–20 Hz) the position of up to 50 markers with respect to the RT system isocenter. The specific characteristic of the system is its capability to separately track groups of markers assigned to different monitoring: 1 marker for patient positioning with respect to the isocenter, most of the markers for the patient's posture, and residual markers for

breathing. The system can therefore be used as an RMTS for BH or gated treatments.

A different approach has been followed by Schaller and colleagues,[67] who proposed time-of-flight (TOF) technology to acquire, in real time and by using a single special camera, a multidimensional respiratory signal from a 3D surface reconstruction of the patient's chest and abdomen (**Fig. 5**). A TOF camera is a device able to detect, in real time, the 3D surface of objects, and comprises 2 main components: an active illuminator and an image sensor. The illuminator emits an incoherent near-IR light signal. The emission range depends on the modulation frequency of the camera, which in turn defines the wavelength of the emitted signal. The signal is modulated in intensity by a cosine-shaped signal of a specific frequency.

The light emitted by the illuminator is reflected by the patient's surface and detected back by the image sensor. In contrast to conventional CCD cameras, in which each cell of the detection matrix produces only a signal proportional to the incident light (intensity signal), in TOF cameras each pixel of the sensor (a photon-mixing device) is able to simultaneously assess the distance of the reflective point (depth information) as well as the corresponding light intensity. Another interesting characteristic of the TOF cameras is that to be ready and operative they do not require any complex setup or calibration procedure, being all-solid-state systems. The device developed by Schaller and colleagues,[67] interestingly, is also

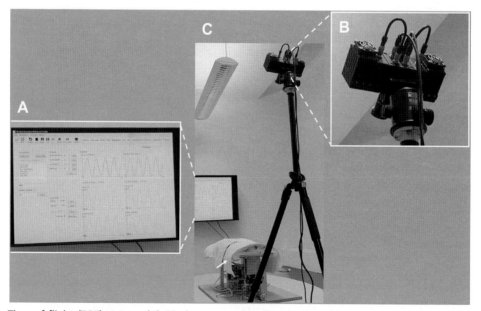

Fig. 5. Time-of-flight (TOF) system. (*A*) Display screen showing the breathing curves as detected by the TOF camera (*B*) from a dynamic breathing phantom (*C, white arrow*).

able to simultaneously and independently describe respiratory signals from different anatomic regions of the body. This capability enables the system to deal with possible changes of the breathing patterns during the evaluation period (eg, from chest breathing to abdominal breathing) allowing determination of the instantaneous type of breathing. To validate the performance of the TOF system, Schaller and colleagues[67] compared its signal to that recorded by the AZ-733V, used as reference. In this test both respiratory signals were synchronized to allow the calculation of the correlation coefficient over different anatomic configurations (eg, thorax, abdomen). The results of the tests showed that an average correlation of 0.91 was obtained for the abdominal region while 0.85 was found over the thorax region. Recently the TOF camera has been also proposed in combination with a rigid registration framework for patient setup and positioning in RT applications.[68]

COACHING TOOLS FOR REGULAR BREATHING

The more regular is the patient's breathing pattern, the higher is the quality of a 4D study. To achieve such a goal it is always important, before starting

a gated acquisition, to perform a check on the ability of the patient to maintain a regular breathing pattern. For patients showing difficulties (eg, patients with pathologies involving the respiratory apparatus), coaching tools may be used.[69,70] Coaching tools are generally provided together with commercial RMTSs and are audio, visual, or both. Audio coaching tools consist of earphones or computer speakers (**Fig. 6**), which play prerecorded audio instructions ("breathe in, breathe out" sequences) prompting the patient to maintain a regular breathing frequency. Audio instructions can be generally calibrated to the breathing characteristics (eg, frequency) of the specific patient and are also used to instruct the patient to perform BH sessions. Audio coaching tools have been shown to be useful in regularizing the breathing frequency of patients; however, it has been verified that in several cases the magnitude and the variability of the breathing signal increases, thus amplifying the range of motion and reducing the gating accuracy.[69]

Video coaching tools consist of screens, such as goggles or computer monitors (see **Fig. 6**), which display to the patient (in real time) his or her breathing signal. Two lines indicating the desired range of respiratory motion are generally

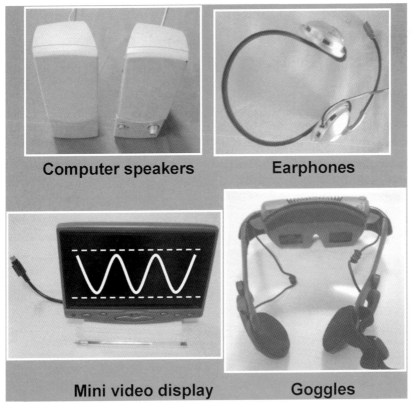

Computer speakers **Earphones**

Mini video display **Goggles**

Fig. 6. Tools needed to perform audio and video coaching.

superimposed on the breathing signal. Visual feedback has been shown to be useful in regularizing the breathing amplitude range, but can induce irregularities in the breathing frequency.[69]

In an attempt to exploit the advantages of both audio and visual coaching systems, tools combining audio and video prompting have been proposed. It has been demonstrated that for patients succeeding in interfacing with these systems, a regular frequency and amplitude can be obtained. However, most patients are not able to accomplish the required double task.

CARDIAC MONITORING AND TRACKING SYSTEMS

The monitoring of cardiac movement is well established and codified. In fact, the cardiac electric activity, which is responsible for the heart beating, is the ideal signal for monitoring and tracking heart contraction and motion. The electrocardiogram (ECG) is therefore the MTS most capable of performing PET and PET/CT cardiac gating. When the sinus-atrial node fires, the electrical impulse that moves toward the atria, causing their contraction, is recorded as a P wave on the ECG. The electrical impulse then moves to the atrioventricular node and successively crosses the ventricles, causing their contraction. The PR interval and the QRS complexes are thus recorded on the ECG. The final return of the ventricles to the resting condition generates the ST segment and the T wave (**Fig. 7**).

When interfaced with the PET or CT imaging system, the ECG provides trigger signals to synchronize the data acquisition to the cardiac cycle. In particular, trigger pulses are usually generated in correspondence to the R peaks. When cardiac gating is performed in prospective mode, data acquisition starts after a specific delay following the R wave (usually after the QRS complex) and then lasts for a defined percentage of the cardiac cycle. When instead gating is performed in retrospective mode, data are collected over the whole cardiac cycle and successively sorted.

To obtain 4D cardiac images free from artifacts, a regular and low cardiac frequency is required. Usually auto-feedback and/or BH maneuvers can help the patient in reducing heart frequency. Otherwise, pharmacologic regulators (eg, β-blockers) must be used.

PET AND PET/CT: ADVANCED RESPIRATORY/ CARDIAC GATING APPLICATIONS AND NEW HARDWARE TECHNOLOGIES

Respiratory and cardiac gating provides images corresponding to different moments of breathing and cardiac cycles. The availability of these gated images enhances the potential of PET and PET/CT in both oncology and cardiology, and opens new scenarios for the diagnostic applications of PET and PET/CT.

In oncology, PET may support CT in the definition of tumor volume in RT treatment planning. In fact, it has been demonstrated that by combining the anatomic information provided by CT with the complementary functional information provided by ^{18}F-labeled 2-deoxy-2-fluoro-D-glucose (^{18}F-FDG) PET, a modification in the RT planning is generally achieved. The modification corresponds to a reduction of the dose distribution volume in the case of an ^{18}F-FDG uptake area smaller than the structural abnormal region, or to an enlargement of the dose distribution volume in the case of PET hypermetabolic areas in regions appearing normal on CT images.[71-73] As an alternative to

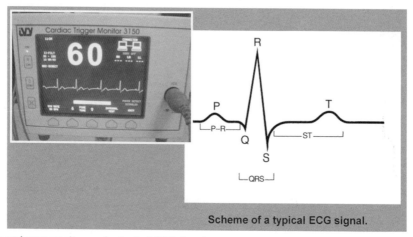

Scheme of a typical ECG signal.

Fig. 7. Cardiac trigger monitor and a typical ECG signal.

^{18}F-FDG, new PET tracers designed to specifically characterize different aspects of the tumor status have been proposed and are currently being evaluated for their potential utility in RT planning: ^{11}C-choline (metabolism), ^{18}F-fluorothymidine (proliferation), ^{64}Cu-diacetyl-bis(N^4-methylthiosemicarbazone) and ^{18}F-fluoromisonidazole (hypoxia), ^{18}F-2-(5-fluoro-pentyl)-2-methyl-malonic acid (apoptosis), and ^{11}C-PD153035 (gene expression for epidermal growth).[74–77] In fact, the future of RT planning lies also in the possibility of defining complex plans incorporating multiple targets in the same volume, based on a molecular imaging characterization of the tumor as a heterogeneous mixture of specific cell populations. The knowledge of the motion trajectory of target and surrounding organs provided by 4D-PET and 4D-PET/CT could also allow to choose the best RT typology for each patient from: (1) standard RT, where the radiation delivery is non-gated and the motion information is used to better circumscribe the treatment volume; (2) gated RT over a specific window of the breathing cycle (eg, end of expiration); and (3) gated RT over the full breathing cycle performed by continuously adapting the dose delivery to the tumor motion.

In cardiology, dual-gating (ie, respiratory and cardiac) PET/CT may further improve the diagnostic power of such imaging techniques to accurately assess heart anatomy and function. PET is in fact a well-recognized tool for quantitative evaluation of cardiac perfusion and metabolism.[78] In particular, PET with ^{18}F-FDG assesses the myocardial metabolism and allows discrimination between irreversible loss of myocardium vitality and partially reversible loss of contractility.[79] Perfusion studies accompanied by kinetic models describing the rate of tracer exchange between the vascular space and the myocardial tissue allow instead quantification of the myocardial blood flow (MBF) and the coronary flow reserve (CFR).[78,80] It has been demonstrated that a joint evaluation of myocardial perfusion and metabolism provides a better understanding of the pathophysiology of ischemic heart diseases.[79] On the anatomic side, multislice CT angiography with 40, 64, and 128 slices enables noninvasive coronary angiographies to be performed, thus facilitating the recognition of stenosis and the measure of the calcification level with a diagnostic accuracy comparable with that of invasive angiography. Therefore PET/CT, provided with a proper tracking/compensation of the heart motion, may become an attractive tool for comprehensive diagnostic evaluation of patients with suspected or proven coronary artery disease as well as other cardiovascular diseases.[81] The acquisition of

PET/CT data in list mode with both respiratory and cardiac synchronization allows the generation of a data set that is variously sorted to obtain: (1) dynamic data for kinetic modeling and quantitative estimation of MBF and CFR; (2) cardiac gating data to assess cardiac volumes, ejection fraction, wall motility, and wall thickening; and (3) respiratory gating data.

Simultaneous cardiac and respiratory gating (dual gating) generates images in which the heart motion is completely frozen.[82–84] These images are used to study coronary arteries for which high spatial resolution is mandatory owing to the small target dimensions. In this regard, one of the most challenging projects is that aimed at detecting coronary plaques prone to rupture.[85–89]

Vulnerable plaques are inflamed and therefore have a high concentration of activated macrophage foam cells around the thin fibrous cap. Angiography is the gold standard for the detection of coronary artery stenosis, but it does not provide information about vessel wall and plaque composition. Magnetic resonance imaging and CT, by contrast, provide information about the plaque structure, but are not specific enough for assessment of plaque vulnerability. ^{18}F-FDG PET has instead been shown to be able to characterize coronary plaques.[86] The intensity of ^{18}F-FDG uptake has in fact been shown to correlate with macrophage density and plaque inflammatory state. Furthermore, recent data suggest that the biological composition and the inflammatory state of an atherosclerotic plaque may be the principal determinants for acute clinical events, more than the degree of stenosis or plaque size. Therefore, gated PET/CT emerges as the combined functional/structural imaging technique with the best potential for the visualization and characterization of coronary atherosclerosis and plaque inflammation.[85,86,88]

The current limitation of the advanced applications discussed here is the low counting statistics level of PET-gated images. In fact, images corresponding to each gate contain a fraction of the total counts, depending on the number of gates into which the study has been divided. In respiratory gating this fraction is generally about 1/6; in dual cardiac/respiratory gating the fraction is much lower, considering that to completely freeze the heart motion the number of respiratory and cardiac gates must be multiplied.[82–84] Excessively low statistics levels force important regularizations in the reconstruction process or important postreconstruction smoothing, which introduce losses in resolution that can negate the gating efforts. Studies trying to optimize the number of gates to achieve a compromise between motion description and image quality have been performed in the literature for both respiratory and cardiac gating.[89–91]

If the main objective of a 4D study is to obtain not a description of the motion but images free from the motion effect, intra-reconstruction or postreconstruction algorithms able to spatially coregister the information contained in each gate to a reference gate can be used. Coregistration may be performed locally (ie, on a small lesion) by using simple rigid spatial transformations,[92,93] or on larger areas (ie, on a whole moving organ) by using more complex spatial transformations. Recently many elastic transformation approaches have been proposed in the literature, with interesting and promising results.[94–101]

If, instead, the objective of a 4D study is to obtain a precise description of the region of interest in each phase of the motion cycle, further efforts to increase the statistics level inside each gate are necessary. All of the current developments in PET technology aim to improve the system sensitivity and therefore move toward the possibility of fully exploiting the 4D approach. One of these improvements consists in adding 1 or more rings of detectors to the standard system configuration. Townsend[102] showed that an increase in the scanner axial field of view (FOV) from 15 to 22 cm results in an increase in the system's sensitivity of about 78%. To further exploit such a possibility, PET tomographs with very wide axial FOV are under simulation/evaluation for the next generation of PET systems.[103] Another improvement regards the research of faster crystal scintillators. Recently introduced lutetium oxyorthosilicate (LSO) and lutetium-yttrium oxyorthosilicate (LYSO) crystals allow achievement of a time resolution of about 500 to 600 picoseconds. The implementation of the TOF technology with LSO and LYSO has demonstrated improvement in the signal-to-noise ratio, in particular in whole-body studies.[104,105] Considering faster scintillators (eg, LuAp, LaBr3) and new photodetectors (eg, SiPMT), a timing resolution of about 300 picoseconds or even better is expected to be obtained in the near future.[106,107] This resolution would theoretically result in an increase in the signal-to-noise ratio of about 2 to 3, which would correspond to a sensitivity gain of about 4 to 8, for sources with diameter between 20 and 35 cm.[108–110]

With the prospect of these improvements in PET-scanner sensitivity, the possibility of performing respiratory gating over the whole region of breathing motion (eg, from the apical region of the lungs down to the whole abdominal region), even for diagnostic whole-body applications, seems realistic in the near future. At present, a 4D-PET/CT protocol generally comprises a conventional whole-body PET/CT acquisition (2–3 min/bed over about 7 beds for a PET tomograph with a 15-cm axial FOV), followed by a respiratory gated 4D-PET/CT acquisition over a single bed (acquisition time of about 8–12 minutes). This kind of protocol leaves completely "ungated" large portions of the body which, conversely, can be affected by respiratory motion. The discussed potential improvements (sensitivity, signal-to-noise ratio) may lead to acquisition times of about 1 to 1.5 minutes for static beds and about 4 to 4.5 minutes for gated beds, thus allowing an increase in the number of gated beds for a total acquisition time compatible with the clinical activity. This kind of 4D-PET whole-body protocol would also require a matched gated CT scan in the region of respiratory gating. In this regard, ultra–low-dose CT scanners, associated with postprocessing of the data and iterative reconstruction algorithms, are under consideration by the research community, in hopes of reducing as much as possible the dose to the patient.[111,112]

SUMMARY

Respiratory/cardiac monitoring and tracking systems synchronize 4D-PET and 4D-PET/CT images to physiologic signals describing the motion of the region under investigation. For the heart beat a standard ECG is commonly used as cardiac MTS, while various respiratory MTSs have been proposed to monitor a surrogate of the true respiratory signal by using a specific technology.

As the detection and compensation of organ motion will be a focal point of the new generation of PET/CT systems, it is expected that for a full assessment of the motion, multidimensional/multitasking MTSs able to simultaneously manage patient, respiratory, and cardiac motions will be specifically designed and implemented for 4D-PET and 4D-PET/CT studies.

These systems will fully satisfy the need for motion management both in oncologic RT planning studies and in diagnostic applications for oncology (detection and compensation of patient/body motion and respiration), cardiology (detection and compensation of patient/chest motion, respiratory motion, and heart motion), and neurology (detection and compensation of patient/head motion).

ACKNOWLEDGMENTS

The authors would like to thank: Dr Fumiko Sakaguchi, Dr Carlo Cavedon, Dr Emanuele Zivelonghi, Dr Schaller C, Dr Pietro Mancosu, Dr Guido

Baroni, and Dr ssa Cristina Garibaldi for providing pictures and technical information about MTSs.

REFERENCES

1. Ter-Pogossian MM, Bergmann SR, Sobel BE. Influence of cardiac and respiratory motion on tomographic reconstructions of the heart: implications for quantitative nuclear cardiology. J Comput Assist Tomogr 1982;6:1148–55.
2. Susskind H, Alderson PO, Dzebolo NN, et al. Effect of respiratory motion on pulmonary activity determinations by positron tomography in dogs. Invest Radiol 1985;20:950–5.
3. Pevsner A, Nehmeh SA, Humm JL, et al. Effect of motion on tracer activity determination in CT attenuation corrected PET images: a lung phantom study. Med Phys 2005;32:2358–62.
4. Park SJ, Ionascu D, Killoran J, et al. Evaluation of the combined effects of target size, respiratory motion and background activity on 3D and 4D PET/CT images. Phys Med Biol 2008;53:3661–79.
5. Townsend DW, Carney JP, Yap JT, et al. PET/CT today and tomorrow. J Nucl Med 2004;45(Suppl 1):4S–14S.
6. Townsend DW. Dual-modality imaging: combining anatomy and function. J Nucl Med 2008;49: 938–55.
7. Osman MM, Cohade C, Nakamoto Y, et al. Respiratory motion artifacts on PET emission images obtained using CT attenuation correction on PET-CT. Eur J Nucl Med Mol Imaging 2003;30:603–6.
8. Mawlawi O, Pan T, Macapinlac HA. PET/CT imaging techniques, considerations, and artifacts. J Thorac Imaging 2006;21:99–110.
9. Nehmeh SA, Erdi YE, Pan T, et al. Four-dimensional (4D) PET/CT imaging of the thorax. Med Phys 2004;31:3179–86.
10. Boucher L, Rodrigue S, Lecomte R, et al. Respiratory gating for 3-dimensional PET of the thorax: feasibility and initial results. J Nucl Med 2004;45: 214–9.
11. Keall PJ, Mageras GS, Balter JM, et al. The management of respiratory motion in radiation oncology report of AAPM Task Group 76. Med Phys 2006;33:3874–900.
12. Bettinardi V, Picchio M, Di Muzio N, et al. PET/CT for radiotherapy: image acquisition and data processing. Q J Nucl Med Mol Imaging 2010;54: 455–75.
13. Gupta T, Beriwal S. PET/CT-guided radiation therapy planning: from present to the future. Indian J Cancer 2010;47:126–33.
14. Ikushima H. Radiation therapy: state of the art and the future. J Med Invest 2010;57:1–11.
15. Lu W, Parikh PJ, Hubenschmidt JP, et al. A comparison between amplitude sorting and phase-angle sorting using external respiratory measurement for 4D CT. Med Phys 2006;33: 2964–74.
16. Dawood M, Büther F, Lang N, et al. Respiratory gating in positron emission tomography: a quantitative comparison of different gating schemes. Med Phys 2007;34:3067–76.
17. Nehmeh SA, Erdi YE, Meirelles GS, et al. Deep-inspiration breath-hold PET/CT of the thorax. J Nucl Med 2007;48:22–6.
18. Fin L, Daouk J, Morvan J, et al. Initial clinical results for breath-hold CT-based processing of respiratory-gated PET acquisitions. Eur J Nucl Med Mol Imaging 2008;35:1971–80.
19. Nehmeh SA, Erdi YE. Respiratory motion in positron emission tomography/computed tomography: a review. Semin Nucl Med 2008;38:167–76.
20. Moorees J, Bezak E. Four dimensional CT imaging: a review of current technologies and modalities. Australas Phys Eng Sci Med 2012;35:9–23.
21. Gierga DP, Brewer J, Sharp GC, et al. The correlation between internal and external markers for abdominal tumors: implications for respiratory gating. Int J Radiat Oncol Biol Phys 2005;61: 1551–8.
22. Ionascu D, Jiang SB, Nishioka S, et al. Internal-external correlation investigations of respiratory induced motion of lung tumors. Med Phys 2007; 34:3893–903.
23. Beddar AS, Kainz K, Briere TM, et al. Correlation between internal fiducial tumor motion and external marker motion for liver tumors imaged with 4D-CT. Int J Radiat Oncol Biol Phys 2007;67:630–8.
24. Kubo HD, Hill BC. Respiration gated radiotherapy treatment: a technical study. Phys Med Biol 1996; 41:83–91.
25. Riedel M. Respiratory motion estimation: tests and comparison of different sensors. IDP—Interdisciplinary Project (Physics). Technische Universität München. Fakultät für Informatik 2006.
26. Zhang T, Keller H, O'Brien MJ, et al. Application of the spirometer in respiratory gated radiotherapy. Med Phys 2003;30:3165–71.
27. D'Souza WD, Kwok Y, Deyoung C, et al. Gated CT imaging using a free-breathing respiration signal from flow-volume spirometry. Med Phys 2005;32: 3641–9.
28. Garcia R, Oozeer R, Le Thanh H, et al. Radiotherapy of lung cancer: the inspiration breath hold with spirometric monitoring. Cancer Radiother 2002;6(1):30–8.
29. Wong JW, Sharpe MB, Jaffray DA, et al. The use of active breathing control (ABC) to reduce margin for breathing motion. Int J Radiat Oncol Biol Phys 1999;44:911–9.
30. Ozhasoglu C, Murphy MJ. Issues in respiratory motion compensation during external-beam

radiotherapy. Int J Radiat Oncol Biol Phys 2002;52: 1389–99.

31. Dawson LA, Brock KK, Kazanjian S, et al. The reproducibility of organ position using active breathing control (ABC) during liver radiotherapy. Int J Radiat Oncol Biol Phys 2001;51:1410–21.

32. Remouchamps VM, Letts N, Vicini FA, et al. Initial clinical experience with moderate deep-inspiration breath hold using an active breathing control device in the treatment of patients with left sided breast cancer using external beam radiation therapy. Int J Radiat Oncol Biol Phys 2003; 56:704–15.

33. Kimura T, Hirokawa Y, Murakami Y, et al. Reproducibility of organ position using voluntary breath-hold method with spirometer for extracranial stereotactic radiotherapy. Int J Radiat Oncol Biol Phys 2004;60:1307–13.

34. Ha J, Perlow D, Yi BY, et al. On the sources of drift in a turbine-based spirometer. Phys Med Biol 2008; 53:4269–83.

35. Martinez-Möller A, Bundschuh R, Riedel M, et al. Comparison of respiratory sensors and its compliance for respiratory gating in emission tomography. J Nucl Med 2007;48(Suppl 2):426P.

36. Noponen T, Kokki T, Lepomaki V, et al. Spirometry based respiratory gating method for cardiac PET and MRI imaging. Nuclear Science Symposium Conference Record, Dresden, Germany, October 19–25, 2008. NSS '08. IEEE pp 4832–34.

37. Vedam SS, Keall PJ, Kini VR, et al. Acquiring a four-dimensional computed tomography dataset using an external respiratory signal. Phys Med Biol 2003;48:45–62.

38. Brandner ED, Wu A, Chen H, et al. Abdominal organ motion measured using 4D CT. Int J Radiat Oncol Biol Phys 2006;65:554–60.

39. Li XA, Stepaniak C, Gore E. Technical and dosimetric aspects of respiratory gating using a pressure-sensor motion monitoring system. Med Phys 2006;33:145–54.

40. Otani Y, Fukuda I, Tsukamoto N, et al. A comparison of the respiratory signals acquired by different respiratory monitoring systems used in respiratory gated radiotherapy. Med Phys 2010; 37:6178–86.

41. Chang Z, Liu T, Cai J, et al. Evaluation of integrated respiratory gating systems on a Novalis Tx system. J Appl Clin Med Phys 2011;12:71–9.

42. Kauweloa KI, Ruan D, Park JC, et al. GateCT™ surface tracking system for respiratory signal reconstruction in 4DCT imaging. Med Phys 2012; 39:492–502.

43. Dunn L, Kron T, Johnston PN, et al. A programmable motion phantom for quality assurance of motion management in radiotherapy. Australas Phys Eng Sci Med 2012;35:93–100.

44. Chi PC, Balter P, Luo D, et al. Relation of external surface to internal tumor motion studied with cine CT. Med Phys 2006;33:3116–23.

45. Carlson SK, Felmlee JP, Bender CE, et al. Intermittent-mode CT fluoroscopy-guided biopsy of the lung or upper abdomen with breath-hold monitoring and feedback: system development and feasibility. Radiology 2003;229:906–12.

46. Carlson SK, Felmlee JP, Bender CE, et al. CT fluoroscopy-guided biopsy of the lung or upper abdomen with a breath-hold monitoring and feedback system: a prospective randomized controlled clinical trial. Radiology 2005;237(2):701–8.

47. Shyn PB, Tatli S, Sainani NI, et al. Minimizing image misregistration during PET/CT-guided percutaneous interventions with monitored breath-hold PET and CT acquisitions. J Vasc Interv Radiol 2011;22:1287–92.

48. Chang G, Chang T, Clark JW Jr, et al. Design and performance of a respiratory amplitude gating device for PET/CT imaging. Med Phys 2010;37: 1408–12.

49. Chang G, Chang T, Pan T, et al. Implementation of an automated respiratory amplitude gating technique for PET/CT: clinical evaluation. J Nucl Med 2010;51:16–24.

50. Nehmeh SA, Haj-Ali AA, Qing C, et al. A novel respiratory tracking system for smart-gated PET acquisition. Med Phys 2011;38:531–8.

51. Meeks SL, Tomé WA, Willoughby TR, et al. Optically guided patient positioning techniques. Semin Radiat Oncol 2005;15:192–201.

52. Wagner TH, Meeks SL, Bova FJ, et al. Optical tracking technology in stereotactic radiation therapy. Med Dosim 2007;32:111–20.

53. Verellen D, Soete G, Linthout N, et al. Quality assurance of a system for improved target localization and patient set-up that combines real-time infrared tracking and stereoscopic X-ray imaging. Radiother Oncol 2003;67:129–41.

54. Jin JY, Yin FF, Tenn SE, et al. Use of the BrainLAB ExacTrac X-Ray 6D system in image-guided radiotherapy. Med Dosim 2008;33:124–34.

55. Wurm RE, Erbel S, Schwenkert I, et al. Novalis frameless image-guided noninvasive radiosurgery: initial experience. Neurosurgery 2008;62:A11–7 [discussion: A17–8].

56. Verellen D, Depuydt T, Gevaert T, et al. Gating and tracking, 4D in thoracic tumours. Cancer Radiother 2010;14:446–54.

57. Yan H, Yin FF, Kim JH. A phantom study on the positioning accuracy of the Novalis Body system. Med Phys 2003;30:3052–60.

58. Spadea MF, Tagaste B, Riboldi M, et al. Intra-fraction setup variability: IR optical localization vs. X-ray imaging in a hypofractionated patient population. Radiat Oncol 2011;6:38.

59. Tagaste B, Riboldi M, Spadea MF, et al. Comparison between infrared optical and stereoscopic X-ray technologies for patient setup in image guided stereotactic radiotherapy. Int J Radiat Oncol Biol Phys 2012;82:1706–14.

60. Spadea MF, Baroni G, Gierga DP, et al. Evaluation and commissioning of a surface based system for respiratory sensing in 4D CT. J Appl Clin Med Phys 2011;12:162–9.

61. Schaerer J, Fassi A, Riboldi M, et al. Multi-dimensional respiratory motion tracking from markerless optical surface imaging based on deformable mesh registration. Phys Med Biol 2012;57:357–73.

62. Vásquez AC, Runz A, Echner G, et al. Comparison of two respiration monitoring systems for 4D imaging with a Siemens CT using a new dynamic breathing phantom. Phys Med Biol 2012;57:N131–43.

63. Baroni G, Ferrigno G, Orecchia R, et al. Real-time three-dimensional motion analysis for patient positioning verification. Radiother Oncol 2000;54:21–7.

64. Gianoli C, Riboldi M, Spadea MF, et al. A multiple points method for 4D CT image sorting. Med Phys 2011;38:656–67.

65. Xia J, Siochi RA. A real-time respiratory motion monitoring system using KINECT: proof of concept. Med Phys 2012;39:2682–5.

66. Lyatskaya Y, Lu HM, Chin L. Performance and characteristics of an IR localizing system for radiation therapy. J Appl Clin Med Phys 2006;7:18–37.

67. Schaller C, Penne J, Hornegger J. Time-of-flight sensor for respiratory motion gating. Med Phys 2008;35:3090–3.

68. Placht S, Stancanello J, Schaller C, et al. Fast time-of-flight camera based surface registration for radiotherapy patient positioning. Med Phys 2012;39:4–17.

69. Kini VR, Vedam SS, Keall PJ, et al. Patient training in respiratory-gated radiotherapy. Med Dosim 2003;28:7–11.

70. Cui G, Gopalan S, Yamamoto T, et al. Commissioning and quality assurance for a respiratory training system based on audiovisual biofeedback. J Appl Clin Med Phys 2010;11:42–56.

71. Ashamalla H, Rafla S, Parikh K, et al. The contribution of integrated PET/CT to the evolving definition of treatment volumes in radiation treatment planning in lung cancer. Int J Radiat Oncol Biol Phys 2005;63:1016–23.

72. Greco C, Rosenzweig K, Cascini GL, et al. Current status of PET/CT for tumour volume definition in radiotherapy treatment planning for non-small cell lung cancer (NSCLC). Lung Cancer 2007;57:125–34.

73. Spratt DE, Diaz R, McElmurray J, et al. Impact of FDG PET/CT on delineation of the gross tumor volume for radiation planning in non-small-cell lung cancer. Clin Nucl Med 2010;35:237–43.

74. Erdi YE. The use of PET for radiotherapy. Curr Med Imag Rev 2007;3:3–16.

75. Macapinlac HA. Clinical applications of positron emission tomography/computed tomography treatment planning. Semin Nucl Med 2008;38:137–40.

76. Zaidi H, Vees H, Wissmeyer M. Molecular PET/CT imaging-guided radiation therapy treatment planning. Acad Radiol 2009;16:1108–33.

77. Bentzen SM, Gregoire V. Molecular imaging-based dose painting: a novel paradigm for radiation therapy prescription. Semin Radiat Oncol 2011;21:101–10.

78. de Jong HW, Lubberink M. Issues in quantification of cardiac PET studies. Eur J Nucl Med Mol Imaging 2007;34:316–9.

79. Ghosh N, Rimoldi OE, Beanlands RS, et al. Assessment of myocardial ischaemia and viability: role of positron emission tomography. Eur Heart J 2010;31:2984–95.

80. DeGrado TR, Bergmann SR, Ng CK, et al. Tracer kinetic modeling in nuclear cardiology. J Nucl Cardiol 2000;7:686–700.

81. Schwaiger M, Ziegler SI, Nekolla SG. PET/CT challenge for the non-invasive diagnosis of coronary artery disease. Eur J Radiol 2010;73:494–503.

82. Martinez-Möller A, Zikic D, Botnar RM, et al. Dual cardiac-respiratory gated PET: implementation and results from a feasibility study. Eur J Nucl Med Mol Imaging 2007;34:1447–54.

83. Teräs M, Kokki T, Durand-Schaefer N, et al. Dual-gated cardiac PET-clinical feasibility study. Eur J Nucl Med Mol Imaging 2010;37:505–16.

84. Kokki T, Sipilä HT, Teräs M, et al. Dual gated PET/CT imaging of small targets of the heart: method description and testing with a dynamic heart phantom. J Nucl Cardiol 2010;17:71–84.

85. Virmani R, Allen BP, Farb A, et al. Pathology of the vulnerable plaque. J Am Coll Cardiol 2006;47:13–8.

86. Chen W, Dilsizian V. (18)F-fluorodeoxyglucose PET imaging of coronary atherosclerosis and plaque inflammation. Curr Cardiol Rep 2010;12:179–84.

87. Pugliese F, Gaemperli O, Kinderlerer AR, et al. Imaging of vascular inflammation with [^{11}C]-PK11195 and positron emission tomography/computed tomography angiography. J Am Coll Cardiol 2010;56:653–61.

88. Joshi F, Rosenbaum D, Bordes S, et al. Vascular imaging with positron emission tomography. J Intern Med 2011;270:99–109.

89. Matter CM, Stuber M, Nahrendorf M. Imaging of the unstable plaque: how far have we got? Eur Heart J 2009;30:2566–74.

90. Bettinardi V, Rapisarda E, Gilardi MC. Number of partitions (gates) needed to obtain motion-free images in a respiratory gated 4D-PET/CT study

as a function of the lesion size and motion displacement. Med Phys 2009;36:5547–58.

91. Dawood M, Büther F, Stegger L, et al. Optimal number of respiratory gates in positron emission tomography: a cardiac patient study. Med Phys 2009;36:1775–84.

92. Livieratos L, Stegger L, Bloomfield PM, et al. Rigid-body transformation of list-mode projection data for respiratory motion correction in cardiac PET. Phys Med Biol 2005;50:3313–22.

93. Bundschuh RA, Martínez-Möller A, Essler M, et al. Local motion correction for lung tumours in PET/CT—first results. Eur J Nucl Med Mol Imaging 2008;35:1981–8.

94. Slomka PJ, Nishina H, Berman DS, et al. "Motion-frozen" display and quantification of myocardial perfusion. J Nucl Med 2004;45:1128–34.

95. Lamare F, Ledesma Carbayo MJ, Cresson T, et al. List-mode-based reconstruction for respiratory motion correction in PET using non-rigid body transformations. Phys Med Biol 2007;52:5187–204.

96. Lamare F, Cresson T, Savean J, et al. Respiratory motion correction for PET oncology applications using affine transformation of list mode data. Phys Med Biol 2007;52:121–40.

97. Rahmim A, Tousset A, Zaidi H. Strategies for motion tracking and correction in PET. PET Clin 2007;2:251–66.

98. Kovalski G, Keidar Z, Frenkel A, et al. Dual "motion-frozen heart" combining respiration and contraction compensation in clinical myocardial perfusion SPECT imaging. J Nucl Cardiol 2009;16:396–404.

99. Qiao F, Pan T, Clark JW Jr, et al. A motion-incorporated reconstruction method for gated PET studies. Phys Med Biol 2006;51:3769–83.

100. Le Meunier L, Slomka PJ, Dey D, et al. Motion frozen (18)F-FDG cardiac PET. J Nucl Cardiol 2011;18:259–66.

101. Gigengack F, Ruthotto L, Burger M, et al. Motion correction in dual gated cardiac PET using mass-preserving image registration. IEEE Trans Med Imaging 2012;31:698–712.

102. Townsend DW. Positron emission tomography/computed tomography. Semin Nucl Med 2008;38:152–66.

103. Poon JK, Dahlbom ML, Moses WW, et al. Optimal whole-body PET scanner configurations for different volumes of LSO scintillator: a simulation study. Phys Med Biol 2012;57:4077–94.

104. Conti M. State of the art and challenges of time-of-flight PET. Phys Med 2009;25:1–11.

105. Lois C, Jakoby BW, Long MJ, et al. An assessment of the impact of incorporating time-of-flight information into clinical PET/CT imaging. J Nucl Med 2012;51:237–45.

106. Schaart DR, Seifert S, Vinke R, et al. LaBr(3):Ce and SiPMs for time-of-flight PET: achieving 100 ps coincidence resolving time. Phys Med Biol 2010;55:N179–89.

107. Daube-Witherspoon ME, Surti S, Perkins A, et al. The imaging performance of a LaBr₃-based PET scanner. Phys Med Biol 2012;55:45–64.

108. Snyder DL, Thomas LJ, Terpogossian MM. A mathematical-model for positron-emission tomography systems having time-of-flight measurements. IEEE Trans Nucl Sci 1981;28:3575–83.

109. Budinger TF. Time-of-flight positron emission tomography—status relative to conventional PET. J Nucl Med 1983;24:73–6.

110. Karp JS, Surti S, Daube-Witherspoon ME, et al. Benefit of time-of-flight in PET: experimental and clinical results. J Nucl Med 2008;49:462–70.

111. Xia T, Alessio AM, De Man B, et al. Ultra-low dose CT attenuation correction for PET/CT. Phys Med Biol 2012;57:309–28.

112. Katsura M, Matsuda I, Akahane M, et al. Model-based iterative reconstruction technique for radiation dose reduction in chest CT: comparison with the adaptive statistical iterative reconstruction technique. Eur Radiol 2012;22:1613–23.

Respiratory Motion Correction Strategies in Thoracic PET-CT Imaging

Sadek A. Nehmeh, PhD

KEYWORDS

- PET-CT • Motion correction

KEY POINTS

- Hybrid PET-CT technology has led to improved sensitivity and specificity as well as enhancement in the value of PET and CT when assessing tumor response to therapy.
- Due to breathing motion, and the difference in time resolutions between PET and CT, motion artifacts and spatial mismatch between the corresponding two image sets are common.
- Correction for the breathing-induced artifacts in PET and CT images represents a particular challenge; some schemes use respiratory-phase data selection to exclude motion artifacts, others have adopted sophisticated software techniques.

INTRODUCTION

The development of PET-CT scanners has allowed robust and synergistic fusion of anatomic and functional information. Combined PET-CT imaging has been shown to yield an increased sensitivity and specificity over any of those of the two individual modalities. This fusion has also resulted in more precise localization and characterization of sites of radiotracer uptake, and has increased the accuracy of diagnosis, staging, restaging, and monitoring of tumor response in different types of cancers.[1–5]

Besides localization, in combined PET-CT, CT images are used to correct for attenuation in the PET images. A spatial matching between the two image sets (ie, PET and CT) is, therefore, vital. However, in particular in the thorax, due to breathing motion and the differences in PET and CT image scan times (6–9 min/bed for PET vs ~15 seconds for CT), misregistration of internal organs between the two modalities is common.[3,6,7] Breathing-induced image artifacts, in both PET and CT, have been reported.[2,4,8] For example, in CT, breathing motion may cause the exclusion of some anatomic structures or repeated scanning of others, resulting in image artifacts, thus affecting the accuracy of diagnosis and target volume definition in radiotherapy.[8] In PET, breathing can result in blurring the target volume, consequently resulting in a reduced measured lesion standard uptake value (SUV).[2–4] Also, because of differences in time resolution between the two modalities, CT may not spatially match the PET images, resulting in an inaccurate attenuation correction in the PET images.[9] Consequently, the target may get mislocalized,[6,10] and the SUV may again be erroneous.[9] Consequently, the use of the change in SUV between pretherapy and posttherapy as a metric to assess tumor response may become unreliable unless PET-CT images are corrected for breathing artifacts. Therefore, correction for breathing induced artifacts in PET-CT images becomes vital.

Many methods have been developed to address respiratory motion correction in PET-CT imaging. This article discusses these together with the different respiratory tracking techniques.

RESPIRATORY-MOTION TRACKING SYSTEMS

Several related techniques have been developed to account for respiratory motion artifacts in PET-CT

Department of Medical Physics, Memorial Sloan-Kettering Cancer Center, New York, NY, USA
E-mail address: nehmehs@mskcc.org

PET Clin 8 (2013) 29–36
http://dx.doi.org/10.1016/j.cpet.2012.10.004
1556-8598/13/$ – see front matter © 2013 Elsevier Inc. All rights reserved.

imaging. For this purpose, a large number of respiratory monitoring systems to track the breathing motion[11] and assist in performing four-dimensional (4D) radiotherapy, 4D CT, 4D cone-beam CT, 4D PET, and breath-hold (BH) PET-CT have been investigated. Most famous of these are

1. Pressure sensor, which correlates the change in stress during breathing by means of a load cell placed inside an elastic belt fastened around the patient's abdomen or thorax.[12–15]
2. Spirometer, which correlates the breathing motion to the air flow to and from the lungs using an air tube placed in the nose or mouth of the patient.[12,15–18]
3. Temperature sensor, which correlates the breathing motion to the difference in the air temperature flowing into and out of the lungs of the patient.[19]
4. The Real-Time Position Management (RPM) Respiratory Gating System is probably the most widely used device to track patient's respiratory motion, in particular during gated radiotherapy. RPM technique is based on tracking the vertical motion of reflective fiducial markers (FMs), placed on the abdomen of the patient, using an infrared camera.[3] The RPM setup for 4D PET-CT is shown in **Fig. 1**. The RPM has been widely implemented in gated radiotherapy applications of lung,[20–23] respiratory-gated CT,[1,24] and 4D CT,[1,25,26] as well as respiratory-gated PET imaging.[2–4] **Fig. 1** shows the RPM setup during 4D PET-CT acquisition.
5. The three-dimensional respiratory tracking system (3D RTS) is an in-house openCV application that was specifically developed to track the breathing motion during 4D PET-CT imaging.[27] 3D RTS uses a camcorder (or webcam) and an edge detection technique to track simultaneously the two-dimensional (2D) motion of multiple FMs placed on the thorax of the patient at a rate of 30 frames per second. There are two major advantages of 3D RTS over RPM. First, 3D RTS uses a standard digital camera to monitor the motion of the external FM's camera, such as web cameras, personal camcorder, and so forth (RPM uses an infrared camera), making the tracking system robust and user friendly. Second, it allows selective acquisition of PET data corresponding to only one breathing (eg, end expiration). This option that is, to the author's knowledge, unique to this device. **Fig. 2** shows the 3D RTS setup for respiratory gated PET-CT. A mini wireless camera has been used to monitor the motion of the FM's.

With the exception of the spirometer and the temperature sensor, the aforementioned systems track the respiratory signal through the measurement of the displacement of an FM placed on the abdomen of the patient. Even though such signal has been shown to correlate with internal organ motion, spirometer, which correlates with lung-volume changes, may be the most accurate. However, it is generally less well-tolerated by patients than the other systems over the long duration of typical PET emission image acquisitions. For BH PET-CT, 3D RTS may be the only device that enables such application in PET-CT imaging.

RESPIRATORY MOTION ARTIFACTS IN PET-CT

In CT images, breathing-induced artifacts are mainly due to the dynamic interaction between transaxial image acquisition and the asynchronous

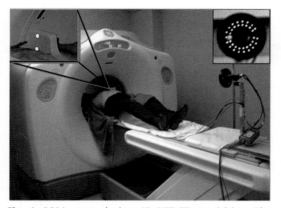

Fig. 1. RPM setup during 4D PET-CT acquisition. The RPM tracks two infrared reflective markers located on the anterior chest surface (*top left*) using an IR video camera (*top right*).

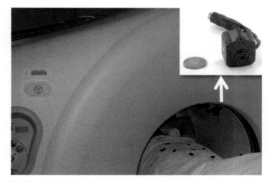

Fig. 2. 3D RTS setup inside the PET-CT gantry during 4D acquisition. 3D RTS uses a miniature wireless camera (*top right*) to simultaneously track the 2D motion of multiple FMs (black markers on the patient's thorax).

motion of tumor and normal tissue.[8] Commonly observed artifacts include distortion of the dome of the liver at the lung-diaphragm interface, splitting of a tumor into multiple distinct parts, out-of-order shuffling of the transaxial slices, and creation of discontinuities in the diaphragm-lung interface.[8] Due to the long acquisition time per bed position (3–7 minutes), PET images are time-averaged over many breathing cycles (average breathing period is 5 seconds). This results in the blurring of the target volume[4,10,28] and reduces the apparent radiotracer uptake.[2,4]

In hybrid PET-CT, respiratory motion can result in hybrid motion artifacts, primarily due to the temporal mismatch between PET images and the corresponding CT-based attenuation map.

A common artifact due to the temporospatial mismatch between PET and CT is the mislocalization of lesions at the border of two organs.[6,10] **Fig. 3** illustrates such an artifact where a liver lesion was incorrectly localized in the lower lung lobe in the PET images.[10] This same lesion was confirmed to reside in the liver for PET images reconstructed without CT-based attenuation correction.[6]

The temporospatial mismatch between PET and CT images can also result in an increased uncertainty in the apparent tumor SUV due to the use of a nonspatially matching CT image set to correct for attenuation in the PET images. Erdi and colleagues[9] showed dependence of the measured tumor SUV on the breathing phase at which CT images were acquired. **Fig. 4** illustrates this effect for a PET lung lesion, where the same PET data set was corrected for attenuation using one 4D CT image set (ie, corresponding to one breathing phase) at a time. Results showed an uncertainty as large as 24% in SUV due to PET-CT mismatch.

CORRECTION FOR BREATHING ARTIFACTS IN PET-CT

As was described previously, respiratory motion can result in mislocalization of the tumor, a reduction in its SUV, and an overestimation of its volume. Attempts to improve the PET to CT coregistration focused on averaging the CT images over multiple breathing phases, thus matching the PET spatial resolution.[29] Even though such an approach improves the PET-CT spatial matching and, therefore, the attenuation correction, it neither reduces image blurring due to breathing motion, nor corrects for the reduction in lesion, detectability, SUV, or target-to-background ratio. In contrast, other algorithms focused on, first, accounting for breathing motion in both PET and CT images and, then, matching those image sets from both modalities based on their corresponding breathing phases.[3,10] Such approaches enable improved PET-CT spatial matching, lesion contrast, and quantitation, as well as image signal-to-noise ratio (SNR). Five such motion correction strategies are described herein.

4D PET-CT

In 4D PET-CT, in which CT is used for attenuation correction and lesion localization, both CT and PET data are acquired simultaneously with the corresponding respiratory motion (ie, in 4D mode). The 4D CT images must, therefore, spatially match the 4D PET images on a phase-by-phase basis. One

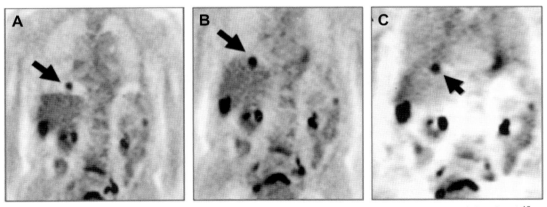

Fig. 3. Mislocalization of liver lesion due to temporal mismatch between PET and CT images. (*A*) A focal [18]FDG uptake in the lower lobe of the right lung appears in the PET with CT attenuation-corrected images. (*B*) The same lesion appears in the liver when PET images were corrected for attenuation using [68]Ge transmission rod sources. (*C*) The finding in (*B*) was confirmed in the nonattenuation corrected PET images. (*Data from* Sarikaya I, Yeung HW, Erdi Y, et al. Respiratory artifact causing malpositioning of liver dome lesion in right lower lung. Clin Nucl Med 2003;28(11):943–4.)

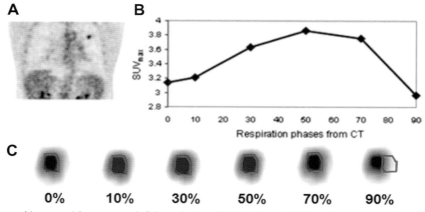

A

B

C

0%   10%   30%   50%   70%   90%

Fig. 4. (*A*) Coronal image with an upper-left lung lesion. (*B*) Variation in SUV_{max} due to correcting for attenuation in the PET images using CT data acquired at different phases within the breathing cycle. (*C*) Cross-sections of PET lesion reconstructed with different phase CTAC. The same threshold window is used for all PET images. The lesion boundary is drawn on the 0% phase and copied onto other phases. At the 90% phase, 9-mm displacement of the region of interest can clearly be seen. (*From* Erdi YE, Nehmeh SA, Pan T, et al. The CT motion quantitation of lung lesions and its impact on PET-measured SUVs. J Nucl Med 2004;45(8):1287–92; with permission.)

method of 4D CT uses a "step-and-shoot" technique (CT images are acquired in cine mode) that acquires repeated axial CT images for a specified period of time, at each table position ($\sim$10 mm).[1] For example, Nehmeh and colleagues[3] used a "shoot" period (cine duration) of one breathing period plus 1 second, a table increment (cine CT axial field of view) of 10 mm (4 × 2.5 mm slice thickness), and an x-ray tube speed of two rotations per second with a cine interval between images of 0.45 seconds (ie, an overlap between consecutive images equivalent to 0.05 seconds of data). To correlate each of the 4D CT images with the corresponding breathing phase, the corresponding respiratory signal will be recorded simultaneously, for example, using the RPM system.[3] During 4D CT acquisition, the RPM system records the state of a transistor-transistor logic "x-ray ON" signal from the CT scanner indicating the time of acquisition of the CT data, thus allowing time-stamping of each of the CT images for retrospective image selection.[1] The 4D CT images are then binned according to the breathing phase based on the RPM respiratory signal, as illustrated in **Fig. 5**.[1]

Likewise, 4D PET data are acquired in correlation with the breathing motion. 4D PET data are acquired in gated mode (similar to cardiac gating), in which data corresponding to each breathing cycle are split into time bins (typically 8 to 10 bins), the width of which is predefined by the user. The data acquisition for each cycle is initialized by a trigger generated by the respiratory tracking device at a user-defined phase or amplitude of the breathing cycle. This trigger is then fed into the PET scanner to initiate

the data collection cycle (ie, into the first bin). The resulting bins' images each corresponds to one breathing phase of the breathing cycle, thus revealing the time-dependence of the gated PET data. Gated PET data are typically acquired for at least 1 minute per bin, compared with 3 minutes per bed in a standard clinical setting (ie, for a total of 10 min/PET bed; $\sim$15 cm), to preserve a relatively acceptable SNR. Consequently, 4D PET images suffer from poorer count rate statistics and, therefore, are characterized by increased noise level and reduced SNR. Finally, the 4D CT images are binned retrospectively at phases matching those of the 4D PET ones, and each of the 4D PET bins is corrected for attenuation with the phase-matched CT image set. In a study that included four subjects with non–small cell lung carcinoma, 4D PET-CT improved PET-CT lesion coregistration by as much as 41%, reduced the PET target volume by up to 42%, and increased lesion SUV by up to 16%, as a result of breathing motion correction.[3] A 4D PET-CT example is illustrated in **Fig. 6**.

Unfortunately, the prolonged time to acquire data from 4D PET-CT, together with the reduced SNR and the long postprocessing time, has limited the widespread clinical use of 4D PET-CT. This has led to the development of more robust approaches (see later discussion).

DEEP-INSPIRATION BH PET-CT

Due to the fast acquisition time ($\sim$16 seconds to image the thorax), BH CT has been well-established in clinical practice for CT image

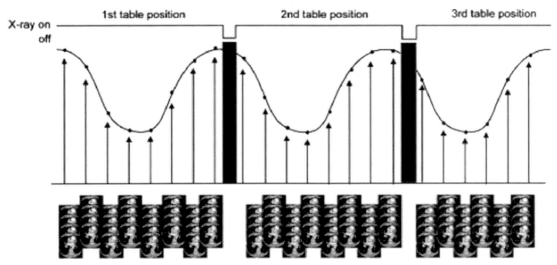

Fig. 5. Data acquisition and retrospective sorting in 4D CT [1]. The "x-ray on" duration during each step of data acquisition is greater than or equal to the average breathing cycle plus the duration of data acquisition for an image reconstruction. The dots on the respiratory signal trace represent the midscan time of the CT image reconstructions. Each dot represents four image reconstructions on a 4-slice CT. There is an "x-ray off" period for table translation from one position to the next position.

acquisition for diagnostic and radiation treatment planning purposes. However, in the case of PET, and because of the long acquisition time per bed position (~3 min/bed), acquiring data in one single breath hold is not possible. Instead, a novel PET data acquisition protocol, assisted by an in-house respiratory tracking device, has been developed to repeatedly and selectively acquire PET data at only the BH CT–matching breathing amplitude, for a total BH PET acquisition time equivalent to the clinical one (ie, 3 min/bed).[30] Nehmeh and colleagues[10] and Meirelles and colleagues[31] showed an increase in lesion SUV by as much as 83% and an improved spatial matching between PET and CT by as much as 50% using BH PET-CT versus standard free-breathing (FB) PET-CT. In a prospective study, Meirelles and colleagues[31] also showed increased lesion detectability with deep-inspiration BH (DIBH) CT over FB CT (on average, 2.2 additional nodules per patient were identified on the DIBH-CT images compared with FB images, especially nodules smaller than 0.5 cm). DIBH CT also allowed more precise localization and characterization of pulmonary lesions than FB CT allowed.[31] Moreover, DIBH PET-CT reduced misregistration between PET and CT caused by internal motion.[10,31] In one case, focal fluorodeoxyglucose F 18 (^{18}F-FDG) uptake apparently localized to the lung on conventional PET-CT was shown to actually represent a rib metastasis on BH PET-CT (**Fig. 7**).[10] This finding was confirmed in CT images. Previous studies showed BH PET-CT to be more robust and to have an improved SNR compared with 4D PET-CT.[10,30]

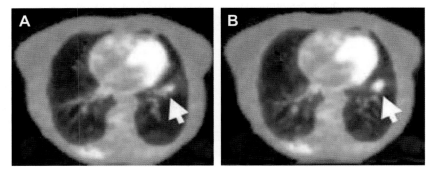

Fig. 6. A transaxial fused PET-CT slice through a patient's lesion as it appears (A) in the nongated acquisition and (B) in the 4D PET-CT study. (From Nehmeh SA, Erdi YE, Pan T, et al. Four-dimensional (4D) PET-CT imaging of the thorax. Med Phys 2004;31(12):3179–86.)

REGISTRATION OF GATED-PET IMAGES

Even though 4D PET-CT results in an improved PET-CT coregistration and lesion contrast,[2–4] it suffers from the reduction in the SNR compared with the clinical PET images owing to the shorter equivalent acquisition time per gated-PET image bin (1 min/bed vs 3 min/bed).[3] One way to improve the SNR in gated-PET images is to, retrospectively, nonrigidly register the gated-PET images from different time bins and, therefore, improve the image quality. For example, Thorndyke and colleagues[32] investigated a B-spline–based deformable registration model for that purpose. This approach enabled a reduction in the respiratory-induced blurring, increase of the SNR, and improvement of the temporal matching between PET and CT image sets.[32–34]

IMAGE RECONSTRUCTION-INTEGRATED MOTION CORRECTION

A more robust approach to correct for respiratory motion in PET images is to incorporate motion information within the reconstruction process to deduce motion-free images. In this scheme, patient-specific motion is extracted from the 4D CT data. Then, using a deformable registration model, with the assumption that 4D PET and 4D CT are both acquired under normal breathing cycles, gated-PET data bins are registered in the sinogram space. This motion-correction technique enabled improved SNR and quantitation of the radiotracer uptake within the tumor.[34,35]

MR-BASED MOTION CORRECTION IN HYBRID PET-MR

The newly emerging simultaneous PET-MR imaging technology allows concordant acquisition of both PET and MR signals, thus providing an improved spatial and temporal alignment between the two modalities. Using tagged-MR imaging acquisition, motion tracking in the phase domain can be performed, thus allowing estimates of the nonrigid deformation of biologic tissues during breathing. Motion fields are then estimated in the

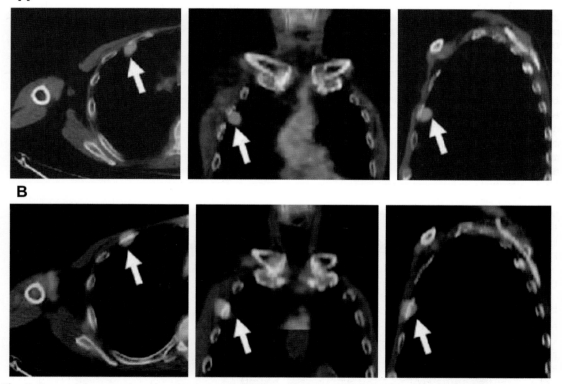

Fig. 7. Transaxial, coronal, and sagittal views of (*A*) standard- and (*B*) DIBH-fused PET and CT images. Arrows point to a lesion in a rib, based on CT images. The PET lesion appears partially in lung in the FB images; only marginally matching the CT lesion because of respiratory motion. DIBH resulted in improved coregistration between PET and CT, and in improved lesion localization. (*From* Nehmeh SA, Erdi YE, Meirelles GS, et al. Deep-inspiration breath-hold PET-CT of the thorax. J Nucl Med 2007;48(1):22–6; with permission.)

system matrix of the PET reconstruction algorithm formulated both for sinogram and list-mode data representations, thus allowing the incorporation of all detected coincidences into one single motion-free image set.[36] This approach yields increased lesion detectability and contrast, as well as SNR, while reducing the total acquisition time many-fold compared with gated-PET acquisition.[36,37] MR-based motion correction in PET images has the potential to allow accurate PET motion correction without increasing the radiation dose, which is a major advantage over PET-CT.[36,37]

SUMMARY

In this article, strategies to correct for respiratory motion in PET-CT images have been summarized. Each has advantages and disadvantages, and the optimum clinical approach remains to be determined. 4D CT may be considered as a driving tool for respiratory gating, especially in a reconstruction-integrated motion-correction approach in which internal organ motion is estimated from 4D CT images.[35] The main concern with 4D CT, however, remains the increased radiation dose compared with conventional CT scans. Besides, irregular breathing makes 4D CT very challenging and can result in major uncertainties.[38] 4D CT can be very useful in radiotherapy planning when assessing the extent of tumor motion. In diagnostic CT, however, the standard practice is to acquire CT images in BH status at end-inspiration to expand the lungs and, therefore, improve the image quality and lesion detectability of the CT images, as was shown by Meirelles and colleagues.[31] Likewise, Nehmeh and colleagues[10,30] and Meirelles and colleagues[31] demonstrated the feasibility of acquiring BH PET images by selectively acquiring PET data corresponding to end-inspiration. BH PET-CT has been shown to have major advantages over 4D PET-CT, particularly in terms of dose, shorter acquisition and postprocessing times, and improved PET-CT coregistration and SNR. However, an improved diagnostic value of BH PET over FB PET, which is the standard clinical acquisition, is yet to be shown.

There have been many attempts to combine PET data from the different gated bins on image space or sinogram and/or list-mode space to improve the SNR.[35–37,39] Klein and colleagues[40] applied their algorithm to high-statistics PET images of the heart. However, for other moving organs, registering gated PET bins may not be accurate because of low statistics. Therefore, the transformation matrices will need to be deduced from 4D CT data, which is a disadvantage that results in increased patient exposure.

In summary, DIBH acquisition seems to be the most robust technique to correct for breathing motion in PET and CT images simultaneously. Compared with 4D PET-CT and software-based corrections, DIBH PET-CT has the advantage of restricting the CT acquisition to the most diagnostically reliable breathing phase (ie, end-inspiration), thus reducing the patient's dose. With the use of 3D RTS developed by Nehmeh and colleagues,[27] PET data can be selectively acquired at end-inspiration with minimum user interference. Besides, DIBH PET-CT acquisition will not require add any postprocessing to what is normally performed in the standard clinical practice. The diagnostic value of end-inspiration PET versus any other breathing phase (eg, end inspiration) is yet to be determined.

Finally, many techniques have been developed to correct for breathing-induced artifacts in the PET-CT images. To the author's knowledge, all previous studies showed the value of motion-correction in improving the image quality and quantitation in PET-CT. Rigorous comparison of image quality and quantitative accuracy among the motion-correction methods discussed remains to be done. Also, whether those improvements make any difference in the final diagnosis and/or patient management compared with non-corrected images is still to be investigated. Studies aiming to evaluate the diagnostic value of motion-free PET-CT images of lung are currently being conducted.

REFERENCES

1. Pan T, Lee TY, Rietzel E, et al. 4D-CT imaging of a volume influenced by respiratory motion on multislice CT. Med Phys 2004;31(2):333–40.
2. Nehmeh SA, Erdi YE, Ling CC, et al. Effect of respiratory gating on reducing lung motion artifacts in PET imaging of lung cancer. Med Phys 2002;29(3): 366–71.
3. Nehmeh SA, Erdi YE, Pan T, et al. Four-dimensional (4D) PET/CT imaging of the thorax. Med Phys 2004; 31(12):3179–86.
4. Nehmeh SA, Erdi YE, Ling CC, et al. Effect of respiratory gating on quantifying PET images of lung cancer. J Nucl Med 2002;43(7):876–81.
5. Dawood M, Lang N, Jiang X, et al. Lung motion correction on respiratory gated 3-D PET/CT images. IEEE Trans Med Imaging 2006;25(4):476–85.
6. Sarikaya I, Yeung HW, Erdi Y, et al. Respiratory artifact causing malpositioning of liver dome lesion in right lower lung. Clin Nucl Med 2003;28(11):943–4.
7. Beyer T, Antoch G, Muller S, et al. Acquisition protocol considerations for combined PET/CT imaging. J Nucl Med 2004;45(Suppl 1):25S–35S.

8. Rietzel E, Pan T, Chen GT. Four-dimensional computed tomography: image formation and clinical protocol. Med Phys 2005;32(4):874–89.

9. Erdi YE, Nehmeh SA, Pan T, et al. The CT motion quantitation of lung lesions and its impact on PET-measured SUVs. J Nucl Med 2004;45(8):1287–92.

10. Nehmeh SA, Erdi YE, Meirelles GS, et al. Deep-inspiration breath-hold PET/CT of the thorax. J Nucl Med 2007;48(1):22–6.

11. Bettinardi V, EDB, Presotto L, et al. Motion tracking hardware and advanced applications in PET and PET/CT. PET Clin 2013;8(2).

12. Kubo HD, Hill BC. Respiration gated radiotherapy treatment: a technical study. Phys Med Biol 1996; 41(1):83–91.

13. Li XA, Stepaniak C, Gore E. Technical and dosimetric aspects of respiratory gating using a pressure-sensor motion monitoring system. Med Phys 2006;33(1):145–54.

14. Dietrich L, Jetter S, Tucking T, et al. Linac-integrated 4D cone beam CT: first experimental results. Phys Med Biol 2006;51(11):2939–52.

15. Martínez-Möller A, BR, Navab N. Comparison of respiratory sensors and its compliance for respiratory gating in emission tomography. J Nucl Med 2007;48(Suppl 2):426.

16. Zhang T, Keller H, O'Brien MJ, et al. Application of the spirometer in respiratory gated radiotherapy. Med Phys 2003;30(12):3165–71.

17. Ozhasoglu C, Murphy MJ. Issues in respiratory motion compensation during external-beam radiotherapy. Int J Radiat Oncol Biol Phys 2002;52(5): 1389–99.

18. Kalender WA, Rienmuller R, Seissler W, et al. Measurement of pulmonary parenchymal attenuation: use of spirometric gating with quantitative CT. Radiology 1990;175(1):265–8.

19. Boucher L, Rodrigue S, Lecomte R, et al. Respiratory gating for 3-dimensional PET of the thorax: feasibility and initial results. J Nucl Med 2004;45(2):214–9.

20. Korreman SS, Juhler-Nottrup T, Boyer AL. Respiratory gated beam delivery cannot facilitate margin reduction, unless combined with respiratory correlated image guidance. Radiother Oncol 2008; 86(1):61–8.

21. Ahmed RS, Shen S, Ove R, et al. Intensity modulation with respiratory gating for radiotherapy of the pleural space. Med Dosim 2007;32(1):16–22.

22. Korreman SS, Pedersen AN, Nottrup TJ, et al. Breathing adapted radiotherapy for breast cancer: comparison of free breathing gating with the breath-hold technique. Radiother Oncol 2005; 76(3):311–8.

23. Yorke E, Rosenzweig KE, Wagman R, et al. Interfractional anatomic variation in patients treated with respiration-gated radiotherapy. J Appl Clin Med Phys 2005;6(2):19–32.

24. Chang JW, Sillanpaa J, Ling CC, et al. Integrating respiratory gating into a megavoltage cone-beam CT system. Med Phys 2006;33(7):2354–61.

25. Pan T, Sun X, Luo D. Improvement of the cine-CT based 4D-CT imaging. Med Phys 2007;34(11):4499–503.

26. Chi PC, Balter P, Luo D, et al. Relation of external surface to internal tumor motion studied with cine CT. Med Phys 2006;33(9):3116–23.

27. Amin Haj-Ali QC, Jaradat HA, Booth P, et al. A miniature and wireless tracking system for respiratory gated PET/CT. J Nucl Med 2009;50(Suppl 2): 1543.

28. Nehmeh SA, Erdi YE, Rosenzweig KE, et al. Reduction of respiratory motion artifacts in PET imaging of lung cancer by respiratory correlated dynamic PET: methodology and comparison with respiratory gated PET. J Nucl Med 2003;44(10):1644–8.

29. Pan TS, Mawlawi C, Nehmeh SA, et al. Attenuation correction of PET images with respiration-averaged CT images in PET/CT. J Nucl Med 2005;46(9):1481–7.

30. Nehmeh SA, Haj-Ali AA, Qing C, et al. A novel respiratory tracking system for smart-gated PET acquisition. Med Phys 2011;38(1):531–8.

31. Meirelles GS, Erdi YE, Nehmeh SA, et al. Deep-inspiration breath-hold PET/CT: clinical findings with a new technique for detection and characterization of thoracic lesions. J Nucl Med 2007;48(5):712–9.

32. Thorndyke B, Schreibmann E, Koong A, et al. Reducing respiratory motion artifacts in positron emission tomography through retrospective stacking. Med Phys 2006;33(7):2632–41.

33. Thorndyke B, Schreibmann E, Maxim P, et al. Enhancing 4D PET through retrospective stacking. Med Phys 2005. AAPM Meeting(TU-D-J-6C-08).

34. Li T, Thorndyke B, Schreibmann E, et al. Model-based image reconstruction for four-dimensional PET. Med Phys 2006;33(5):1288–98.

35. Feng Qiao TP, Clark JW Jr, Mawlawi OR. Compensating respiratory motion in PET image reconstruction using 4D PET/CT. IEEE Nucl Sci Symp Conf Rec 2005;5:2595–8.

36. Chun SY, Reese TG, Ouyang J, et al. MRI-based nonrigid motion correction in simultaneous PET/MRI. J Nucl Med 2012;53(8):1284–91.

37. Guerin B, Cho S, Chun SY, et al. Nonrigid PET motion compensation in the lower abdomen using simultaneous tagged-MRI and PET imaging. Med Phys 2011;38(6):3025–38.

38. Abdelnour AF, Nehmeh SA, Pan T, et al. Phase and amplitude binning for 4D-CT imaging. Phys Med Biol 2007;52(12):3515–29.

39. Thorndyke B, Schreibmann E, Maxim P, et al. Enhancing 4D PET through retrospective stacking. Med Phys 2005;32(6):2096.

40. Klein GJ, Reutter BW, Huesman RH. Four-dimensional affine registration models for respiratory-gated PET. IEEE Trans Nucl Sci 2001;48(3):756–60.

Attenuation Correction Strategies for Positron Emission Tomography/ Computed Tomography and 4-Dimensional Positron Emission Tomography/ Computed Tomography

Tinsu Pan, PhD[a],*, Habib Zaidi, PhD, PD[b,c,d]

KEYWORDS

- Positron emission tomography/computed tomography • Average computed tomography
- 4-dimensional computed tomography • 4-dimensinal positron emission tomography
- 4-dimensional positron emission tomography/computed tomography

KEY POINTS

- Fast helical computed tomography (CT) does not reduce misregistration between the CT and the positron emission tomography (PET) data.
- Average CT matches PET in temporal resolution and improves registration with the PET data.
- Radiation dose of average CT can be as low as less than 1 mSv.
- 4-dimensional CT has been successfully adopted in radiation therapy treatment planning.
- List-mode data acquisition improves the work flow of 4-dimensional PET.
- More promising approaches are being explored in clinical and research settings.

INTRODUCTION

Although the idea of positron emission tomography/computed tomography (PET/CT) emerged in 1993, with the first prototype designed in 1998,[1] it was not until 2001 when the first commercial PET/CT scanner became available.[2] Before the introduction of PET/CT technology, the CT and the PET data were acquired in 2 different scanners. Fusion of the PET and CT data was performed using software techniques.[3,4] Registration of the PET and CT data was relatively accurate for brain studies using rigid transformation but not very successful for the other regions of the body, in particular in the thorax and the abdomen, due to the difficulty of repositioning the patient in 2 separate sessions and the nonrigid nature of the organs.

This work was supported by the Swiss National Science Foundation under grant SNSF 31003A-135576, Geneva Cancer League and the Indo-Swiss Joint Research Programme ISJRP 138866.
Conflict of Interest Notification: Dr Tinsu Pan is the owner of Texas Medical Imaging Consultants, LLC.
a Department of Imaging Physics, MD Anderson Cancer Center, The University of Texas, Unit 1352, 1515 Holcome Boulevard, Houston, TX 77030, USA; b Division of Nuclear Medicine and Molecular Imaging, Geneva University Hospital, CH-1211 Geneva, Switzerland; c Geneva Neuroscience Center, Geneva University, CH-1211 Geneva, Switzerland; d Department of Nuclear Medicine and Molecular Imaging, University Medical Center Groningen, University of Groningen, 9700 RB Groningen, Netherlands
* Corresponding author.
E-mail address: tpan@mdanderson.org

PET Clin 8 (2013) 37–50
http://dx.doi.org/10.1016/j.cpet.2012.09.009
1556-8598/13/$ – see front matter © 2013 Elsevier Inc. All rights reserved.

The advent of PET/CT scanners has made possible for the first time that a single imaging table transporting the patient between PET and CT to hardware fuse the PET and CT data sets. It has been shown that hardware fusion is more accurate than software fusion in clinical diagnosis, staging and restaging of many cancer types such as tumor infiltration of adjacent structures that could not be conclusively assessed using the separate CT and PET data.[5–7] There are over 3000 PET/CT scanners installed worldwide,[8,9] and stand-alone PET scanners have not been in production since 2005.[10] Fluorodeoxyglucose (^{18}F-FDG) is the major pharmaceutical agent in PET/CT, and it has been approved in the United States for diagnosis, staging, and restaging of lung cancer, colorectal cancer, esophageal cancer, head and neck cancer, lymphoma, and melanoma since 1998.[11] In addition, PET/CT has been approved for staging and re-staging and for therapeutic monitoring of breast cancer.

The application of PET/CT is mainly in oncology with ^{18}F-FDG[12–16] and in cardiology with [82]Rb or ^{13}N-NH$_3$ for myocardial perfusion imaging.[17] PET/CT also plays an important role in biologically guided radiation therapy[18,19] and treatment response assessment.[20,21] Integration of functional PET data with anatomic CT data should be a standard in radiation therapy.[14,22] However, it remains a challenge to quantify the improvement of simulation with PET/CT over CT in radiation treatment planning, as conclusive clinical data are not yet available. Early studies have found PET/CT has advantages over CT in standardization of volume delineation,[23,24] in reduction of the risk for geometric misses,[25] and in minimization of radiation dose to the nontarget organs.[13,15,26] Use of PET/CT is expected to grow as more molecular targeted imaging agents are being developed.[27,28]

There are challenges in PET/CT imaging. PET needs CT data for tumor localization, attenuation correction, and quantification. The use of CT-based attenuation correction (CT-AC) for PET data has greatly improved the throughput of PET/CT scan and patient comfort when a CT scan of 100 cm can be performed in less than 20 seconds on a 16-slice PET/CT and less than 10 seconds on a 64-slice PET/CT. In general, 16-slice CT is sufficient for tumor imaging, and 64-slice CT is required for coronary artery imaging. The progress in CT-AC methodology has been immense in the last few years, the main opportunities arising from the development of both optimized scanning protocols and innovative image processing algorithms. However, the use of CT images for attenuation correction of PET data is known to produce artifacts in the resulting PET images in some cases.[29,30] This includes artifacts resulting from the polychromaticity of x-ray photons and resulting beam hardening, misregistration between emission and transmission data, the use of contrast-enhanced CT, truncation resulting from the limited field-of-view of CT, the presence of metallic objects, and artifacts arising from x-ray scatter in CT images.[31]

Application of PET/CT in nuclear medicine or radiology is a detection and quantitation task based on standardized uptake value (SUV).[32–34] Physicians can sometimes mentally construct an ideal image even if the images are with artifacts. If the artifacts are not significant, they can simply be read through. Any mismatch between the CT and the PET data in PET/CT may compromise localization and quantification of the PET data. For example, administration of the intravenous contrast in the CT scan before the PET scan may cause artifacts in the attenuation-corrected PET data. The high-attenuation contrast media can cause over-correction of the PET data. This artifact can appear focal and mimic a malignant lymph node in the axilla or supraclavicular area.[35] Patient motion between the CT and the PET scan is another source of artifacts. Registration with the rigid translation and/or rotation of the CT images to match with the PET data may be sufficient to fix the brain images such as those shown in **Fig. 1**. This article will focus on attenuation correction strategies in PET/CT to mitigate the respiration-induced artifacts in PET/CT and 4-dimensional PET/CT, which are more difficult to correct with postprocessing registration software.

CAUSES OF MISREGISTRATION DUE TO RESPIRATORY MOTION

Misregistration between the CT and PET images due to respiratory motion in the thorax and abdomen was reported soon after the first commercial PET/CT was introduced in 2001[36–39] and has been among the most researched topics in PET/CT. It has impact on radiation therapy, which relies on accurate localization of the tumor for targeted treatment. Radiation oncologists cannot reliably plan therapy by assuming the target tumor at a certain location when it is not the case. They may not be familiar with pitfalls associated with PET/CT imaging, and as such, they generally rely on PET/CT images and the diagnosis and staging information provided by nuclear medicine physicians or radiologists to treat their patients. Both the location and extent of tumor are critical to the success of the process.

Myocardial perfusion imaging with PET/CT also relies on accurate quantification of the PET data,

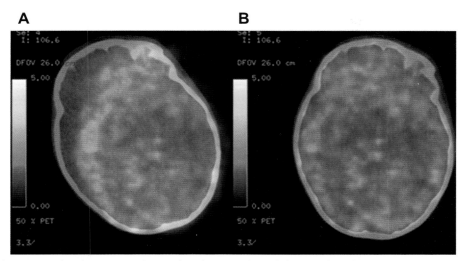

Fig. 1. (*A*) An example of overcorrection and undercorrection of the PET data due to misregistration of the CT and the PET data from the patient motion is shown. (*B*) After applying registration to align the CT and the PET data, improvement in quantification based on the registered PET and CT data is shown.

which depends on accurate registration of CT and PET images for attenuation correction. In general, accurate quantification of the PET images is more critical for myocardial perfusion imaging in cardiology and treatment planning in radiation therapy than for nuclear medicine because of the targeted imaging nature of cardiology and radiation therapy versus whole-body PET imaging in nuclear medicine.

A fast CT scan can cover 100 cm in 10 to 20 seconds, and fast CT gantry rotation can freeze the breathing state in each CT slice. On the other hand, PET takes 2 to 5 minutes to acquire the data of every 15 to 21 cm in the cranial–caudal direction.[40,41] The temporal resolutions of CT and PET are very different: less than 1 second for CT and about 1 respiratory cycle for PET from averaging the PET data of many respiratory cycles. **Fig. 2** shows an example of 2 CT images at the same slice location of 2 different breathing

conditions: free-breathing and deep-inspiration breath-hold. Different breathing states in CT slices and mismatch of the temporal resolution between CT and PET can cause a misalignment of the tumor or the heart position between the CT and the PET data, and compromise quantification of the PET data.[42]

The current design of PET/CT only matches the spatial resolution of the CT and PET data by blurring the CT images so that the spatial resolution of the CT images matches with the spatial resolution of the PET images. There has been no attempt from the manufacturers to match the temporal resolutions of CT and PET for a routine whole-body PET/CT scan. One limitation in PET/CT imaging is that the acquisition time cannot be too long. It is because the patient's arms are normally raised up over the head during data acquisition. In this position, an average person can maintain a still position for about 15 to 30 minutes at maximum.

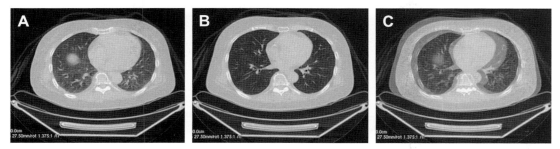

Fig. 2. CT images of the same patient at the same slice location for (*A*) free breathing, (*B*) deep-inspiration breath hold and (*C*) superposition of the 2 CT images in (*A*) and (*B*) to illustrate a potential difference in anatomy between 2 different breathing states.

Mismatch between the CT and the PET data can be identified by a curvilinear white band or photon-penic region near the diaphragm in the PET images (**Fig. 3**). Existence of the white band only suggests a misregistration near the diaphragm and does not mean misregistration at the tumor location. It is possible to have good registration at the tumor location but poor registration at the diaphragm position or vice versa. Note that the heart is always on top of the diaphragm; the problem of misregistration in cardiac PET can be identified more easily in this situation.

Since people spend more time in expiration than in inspiration, the PET data averaged over several minutes are closer to the end-expiration than the end-inspiration. If the CT data are acquired near the end-expiration, then the CT and the PET data may register together better. On the other hand, if the CT data are acquired in or near the end-inspiration, the inflated lungs of inspiration will be larger than the deflated lungs of expiration. The larger area of the inflated lungs in CT renders less attenuation correction in the reconstruction of the PET data near the diaphragm where the inflated lungs push the diaphragm lower in CT than the average diaphragm position in PET. The result is a white band region identified as the misregistered region or the photon-penic region.

FREQUENCY OF MISREGISTRATION

The rate of misregistration can be as high as 68%[43] to 84%.[37] However, it only impacted 2% of diagnosis in the whole-body PET/CT with ^{18}F-FDG[44] but caused false-positive results in 40% of the cardiac PET/CT studies with [82]Rb.[45] In whole-body PET/CT, many lesions may not be close to the diaphragm, where most misregistrations occur; and as such, the task of diagnosis may not be compromised by a misregistration between the CT and the PET data. Since the heart is right above the diaphragm, and diagnosis of a cardiac PET is dependent on accurate quantification of the PET data, a more stringent requirement in registration is needed for the cardiac PET/CT than for whole-body PET/CT. For radiation therapy, there has been a study of 216 patients in quantification and gross tumor volume (GTV) delineation.[43] In this study, 68% had respiratory artifacts, and 10% of the misregistrations could cause an SUV change of over 25%, a threshold indicating a response to therapy.[46] Tumors less than 50 cm³ near the diaphragm could have a change of the centroid tumor location of 2.4 mm, a GTV change of 154% and an SUV change of 21%.

FAST CT DOES NOT REDUCE MISREGISTRATION

It is important to recognize that fast translation of the CT table during a helical CT scan may not eliminate or reduce misregistration between the CT and the PET data. It was suggested that CT images register better between slices if the CT scanner has at least 6 slices.[41] It is true that fast CT gantry rotation helps reduce motion artifacts in each CT slice. However, better registration between slices

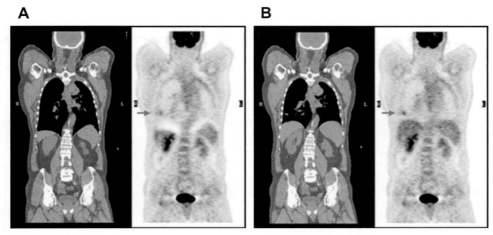

A   **B**

Fig. 3. (*A*) When the CT data have a lower diaphragm position than the PET data, a photo-panic region with an underestimation of FDG uptake in SUV = 2.3 around the diaphragm is shown. (*B*) After correction of the PET data with the average CT data, the photo-penic region disappeared and the SUV of the tumor (pointed by the arrow) increased by 57% from 2.3 to 3.6. (*Reproduced from* Zaidi H, Pan T. Recent advances in hybrid imaging for radiation therapy planning: the cutting edge. PET Clinics 2011;6(2):216; with permission.)

in CT and less motion artifacts in each CT slice do not translate into better registration between the CT and the PET data. Coaching the patient to hold breath at midexpiration during CT acquisition has been suggested.[47] The outcomes were mixed, because coaching patient to hold breath at a certain state during CT data acquisition is not reliable both from the patient and the technologist operating the PET/CT scanner perspectives. In a study of 100 patients coached to hold breath at midexpiration, 50 patient data sets exhibited a misalignment (>1 cm) between the CT and the PET data.[42]

It is clear that as long as the CT scan is conducted when the patient is free breathing, there is always possibility that the CT and the PET data may be misaligned, because some CT slices are taken at inspiration, and some at expiration while the PET data are averaged over several minutes. The distance between 2 end-expiration phases can become longer (or shorter) with a faster (or slower) speed helical CT scan. **Fig. 4** shows an example of CT images taken when the patient was free breathing during a CT scan at the speed of 1.72 cm/s. There were respiratory artifacts on the abdomen and cardiac pulsation artifacts on the heart. These artifacts were not discernible in the

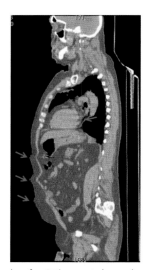

Fig. 4. Example of a CT image taken when the patient was free breathing during a CT scan at the speed of 1.72 cm/s. There were respiratory artifacts (*pointed by three arrows*) on the abdomen and cardiac pulsation artifacts (*pointed by an arrow to the heart*) on the heart. These artifacts were not obvious in each CT slice. Presentation of the artifacts depends on the speed of the helical CT scan and the breathing patterns of the patient during the CT scan. (*Reproduced from* Zaidi H, Pan T. Recent advances in hybrid imaging for radiation therapy planning: the cutting edge. PET Clinics 2011;6(2):212; with permission.)

review of each individual CT slice. By measuring the distance between the adjacent peaks of the respiratory (cardiac pulsation) artifacts and dividing the distance to the table translation speed of the helical CT scan, one can estimate the breathing cycle (the heart rate) of the patient. These artifacts were due to the respiration and the heart beat of the patient. Presentation of the artifacts depends on the speed of the helical CT scan and the breathing patterns of the patient during the fast CT scan.

AVERAGE CT OF LESS THAN 1 mSv REDUCES MISREGISTRATION

Many potential solutions have been suggested to accommodate differences between breathing patterns including retrospective AC using free breathing CT,[48] the use of optimal CT acquisition protocols,[49,50] respiratory averaged CT,[42,51–53,59] interpolated average CT,[54,55] phased CT acquisitions,[56–58] cine CT acquisition,[59] respiratory correlated acquisitions,[60–62] deep-inspiration breath-hold acquisition,[44,63–65] and the use of respiratory-gated PET/CT acquisitions.[66–75]

One approach to improve registration between the CT and the PET data is to bring the temporal resolution of the CT images to that of the PET data.[42] Recognizing the fact that PET is averaged over many breath cycles, a CT image averaged over 1 breath cycle should improve registration between the CT and the PET data. **Fig. 3** shows an example of misregistration between the CT and the PET data, and correction of misregistration with average CT to improve tumor quantification. This concept has also been shown to be effective in attenuation correction of the PET data in cardiac imaging.[51]

Acquiring average CT can be accomplished by scanning at the same slice location over a breath cycle at a high-speed gantry rotation to achieve temporal resolution of less than 1 second for each acquired CT image. The CT images of many phases in a respiratory cycle, mostly free of motion artifacts, are averaged for average CT (**Fig. 5**). The conventional approach using the slow-scan CT of 4 second gantry rotation to generate average CT is ineffective and should be discouraged.[51,76] **Fig. 6** shows a clinical example of the same patient scanned with the slow-scan CT of 4 seconds per gantry rotation and average CT of fast gantry rotation of 0.5 seconds for 4 seconds. The image generated by a slow 4-second gantry had motion artifacts, because the projection data of a slow 4-second CT were inconsistent over 1 revolution of the CT scan. In the approach of using fast gantry rotation for average CT, each CT image was

A

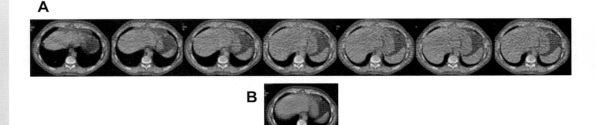

B

Fig. 5. Averaging of the CT images taken at the same slice location over a respiratory cycle in (A) generates the average CT image in (B). Each CT image in (A) was taken at 5 mAs (10 mA and 0.5 second gantry rotation) on the GE Light Speed CT scanner (GE Healthcare, Waukesha, WI).

acquired over a sub-second CT gantry rotation and was without motion artifacts. Averaging over a breath cycle of these high temporal resolution CT images can produce an average CT image with a similar temporal resolution as the PET data.

Cine CT and low-pitch helical CT (pitch <0.1) scans can be adopted to obtain average CT, and both have been used in 4-dimensional CT imaging.[77–79] However, it is not clear whether the setup of 4-dimensional CT imaging primarily for the assessment of tumor motion is ideal for obtaining average CT when most PET/CT scanners are in nuclear medicine and are without the respiratory monitoring device needed for 4-dimensional CT. A practical approach is to acquire average CT without a respiratory monitoring device to improve quantification of the PET data.[51,80] The additional radiation dose for average CT can be less than 1 mSv, and the additional scan time is less than one minute and will not impact the overall scan time of a PET/CT procedure. Selection of optimum parameters for acquiring average CT with cine CT or low-pitch helical CT has been reported.[52]

In terms of temporal resolution, average CT is about 1 respiratory cycle, while the transmission map acquired with rotating rod sources of ^{68}Ge and ^{137}Cs is also about 1 respiratory cycle from averaging of many respiratory cycles. Average CT can be used to approximate the transmission map in terms of temporal resolution. Pan and colleagues[42] demonstrated that registration of the CT and PET data can be improved with average CT in tumor imaging and myocardial perfusion imaging.[51] Papathanassiou and colleagues[81] and Osman and colleagues[37] showed that using the attenuation map from transmission rod sources to correct for the PET images would not produce the curvilinear cold artifacts in the PET data of PET/CT. Transmission rod source is only available in the first-generation PET/CT scanners and not available on the newer PET/CT scanners. The advantages of average CT over transmission rod sources are short acquisition time (1 minutes for CT, and 10 min/15 cm in transmission) and high photon flux and less noisy attenuation maps. The disadvantages are higher radiation dose of less than 1 mSv from average CT than about 0.13 mSv from the transmission rod sources.[82] Radiation therapy has embraced the use of average CT for dose calculation.[83] Since most of

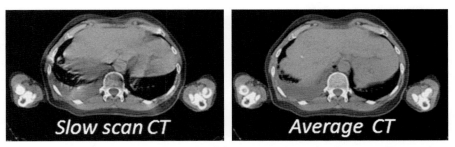

Fig. 6. Comparison of slow-scan CT and average CT of the same patient. The slow-scan CT was taken on a single gantry rotation of 4 seconds, and the average CT was taken from the average of 8 images of 0.5 second gantry rotation for 4 seconds. The artifacts in the slow-scan CT due to reconstruction of the inconsistent CT data in the 4-second scan due to respiration are not in the average CT image. (*Reproduced from* Pan T, Mawlawi O, Luo D, et al. Attenuation correction of PET cardiac data with low-dose average CT in PET/CT. Med Phys 2006;33(10):3937; with permission.)

the new PET/CT scanners are not equipped with transmission rod sources, average CT can serve as an alternative for transmission rod sources. **Fig. 7** shows an example of combining the fast helical CT images and the average CT images of the target tumor area to minimize the area of radiation incurred by the average CT scan. In a whole-body PET/CT examination, the CT images are typically acquired before PET. The technologist can determine if an additional average CT scan is needed when the CT and the PET images of the thorax and the abdomen are available before completion of the PET scan. **Fig. 8** shows an example of average CT improving the registration and quantification of a lymph node. **Fig. 9** shows an example of improvement in the registration and quantification of a lung tumor near the diaphragm and the heart.

Fig. 10 shows an example of misregistration that caused a false-negative diagnosis and a change of the gross target volume for radiation therapy. In the era of image-guided radiation therapy to deliver a very high dose at a great precision, it is very important to pay attention to any misregistration between the CT and the PET images during tumor delineation.

4-DIMENSIONAL PET IMAGING

4-dimensional PET was first developed for cardiac imaging to assess myocardial motion and to obtain ejection fraction 3 decades ago.[84] It was adopted for tumor imaging of the thorax almost a decade ago,[60,66–68] about the same time when 4-dimensional CT was launched.[62,77–79,85] Today, 4-dimensional CT has been accepted as a standard practice in CT imaging of tumor motion for radiation therapy. 4-dimensional PET is still not yet widely accepted as a standard practice. It may be that PET is primarily used for clinical diagnosis and staging, and that a 4-dimensional PET scan is typically conducted after a whole-body PET scan. The total scan time may become too long for any patient to stay still for the 4-dimensional PET imaging.

In 4-dimensional PET, the data are split into several exclusive bins. For example, there can be 8 bins of 500 milliseconds for an average respiratory cycle of 4 seconds. Because of insufficient statistics of photons obtained in PET imaging of 2 to 5 minutes for the selection of 8 bins in each bed location, the duration of a 4-dimensional PET scan has to be over 5 minutes to compensate for the fewer photons recorded in each bin. It may be necessary to scan 2 bed positions if a tumor or the heart is not at the center of the PET detector field of view to compensate for the high sensitivity at the center and the low sensitivity at the edge of the PET detector in 3-dimensional data acquisition without septa.

Image reconstruction of 4-dimensional PET is performed on the data of each bin, and the result is a set of 3-dimensional PET images over a respiratory cycle for assessment of tumor motion and quantification. Even though the number of photons in each bin can be small, resulting in higher noise in

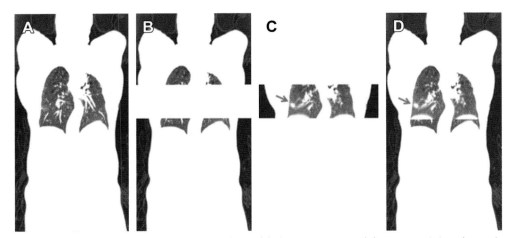

Fig. 7. (A) Conventional CT acquired in free breathing; (B) the CT images in (A) not containing the region containing the tumor; (C) the CT images containing the tumor (*pointed by an arrow*) obtained with average CT; and (D) combination of (B) and (C) to make an image for attenuation correction of the PET data. (*Reproduced from Pan T, Mawlawi O, Nehmeh SA, et al. Attenuation correction of PET images with respiration-averaged CT images in PET/CT. J Nucl Med 2005;46(9):1483; with permission.*)

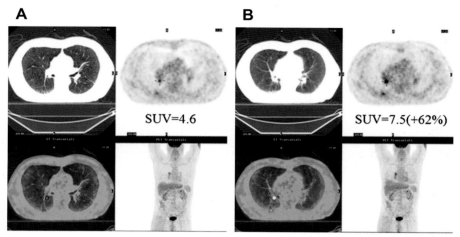

Fig. 8. (*A*) The lymph node shown in PET did not register with the CT and had an SUV of 4.6. (*B*) After attenuation correction with average CT, which registered better with the PET data, the lymph node had an SUV value of 7.5, a 62% increase in SUV. (*Reproduced from* Pan T, Mawlawi O, Nehmeh SA, et al. Attenuation correction of PET images with respiration-averaged CT images in PET/CT. J Nucl Med 2005;46(9):1485; with permission.)

the 4-dimensional PET images,[86] the 4D PET images can potentially be used for accurate assessment of FDG uptake.[68]

Most modern PET/CT scanners are equipped with the list-mode data acquisition, whereby events from each coincidence pair of 511 keV photons can be stored in a list stream for subsequent static, dynamic, or gated reconstruction (**Fig. 11**). List-mode data acquisition can be performed with either cardiac or respiratory triggering during a normal static image acquisition.[87] This functionality offers the capability of retrospectively mapping the coincidence events into multiple phases/bins for the reconstruction of 4-dimensional PET images. PET scanners can be configured to acquire the list-mode data, which can produce prospectively static PET data as a standard data set and retrospectively 4-dimensional PET data to freeze the tumor motion. It is still cumbersome to acquire 4-dimensional PET data due to its prolonged acquisition time. However, it is expected that with the introduction of advanced detector technologies, large detector coverage for higher sensitivity, and incorporation of time-of-flight information in

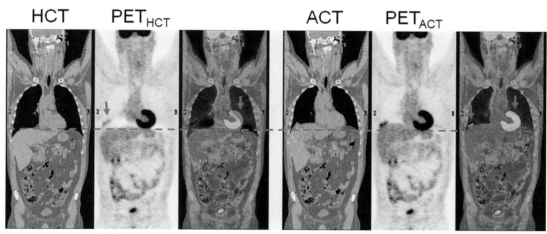

Fig. 9. The standard set of the helical CT (HCT) and the PET data corrected with the HCT is shown in the left panel. Misregistration of the tumor and the heart can be identified and pointed by arrows. Attenuation correction with the average CT (ACT) data is in the right panel. The SUV of the tumor (*pointed by an arrow*) increased from 2.6 to 5.0. The activity in the heart region (*pointed by an arrow*) also increased due to the improved registration of the PET and ACT data.

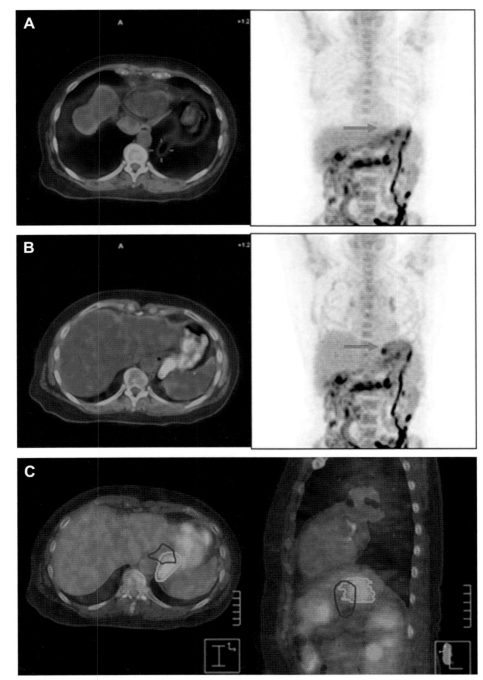

Fig. 10. PET/CT images of a 69 year-old woman with an esophageal tumor after induction chemotherapy. (A) An axial slice of the fused clinical CT and PET image at the level of the esophageal tumor (left) and the PET image in coronal view (right). The diagnosis indicated that the patient had a positive response to the chemotherapy. After removal of the misalignment by average CT, the tumor reappeared in the same PET data set in (B). The arrows point to the tumor location. The gross target volumes drawn in the images of (A) and (B) are shown in blue and in green, respectively, in (C). The patient was treated with the tumor volume in green, and the diagnostic report was corrected by the average CT. (*Reproduced from* Pan T, Mawlawi O. PET/CT in radiation oncology. Med Phys 2008;35(11):4960; with permission.)

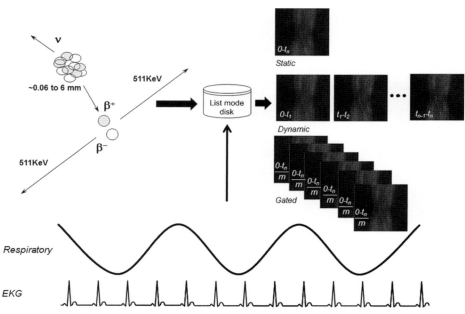

Fig. 11. Schematic diagram of the list-mode data acquisition. The positron coming out of positron emitters such as ^{18}F or ^{82}Rb travels a distance of average 0.06 mm for ^{18}F or 6 mm for ^{82}Rb. The larger the positron energy, the longer the distance it travels. An annihilation event occurs when a positron meets with an electron to emit two 511 keV energy photons and is detected by a pair of PET detectors. List-mode acquisition records the events and the physiologic signal such as the electrocardiogram and/or respiratory signal to guide image reconstruction. Out of the list-mode data acquisition, one can reconstruct the static images of time 0 to t_n, or dynamic images of time 0 to t_1, t_1 to t_2, ..., t_{n-1} to t_n or m gated images of time 0 to t_n. Each picture represents a sinogram for reconstruction.

3-dimensional image reconstruction to better cope with the increased noise from randoms and scatter in 3-dimensional data acquisition. The limitation in acquisition time will be lifted, 4-dimensional PET will become a clinically feasible solution to improve the quantification accuracy of a tumor or the heart in motion.

4-DIMENSIONAL PET/CT IMAGING

4-dimensional CT[77–79] may be needed for accurate quantification of 4-dimensional PET data, as each phase of PET data may need its own CT data for attenuation correction.[68] Four-dimensional CT has found its acceptance in radiation therapy for providing the gated CT images of multiple phases over a respiratory cycle to assist contouring the extent of tumor motion. Four-dimensional CT takes less time in data acquisition than 4-dimensional PET does. It normally takes less than 2 minutes to cover 35 cm in the superior–inferior direction on an 8- or 16-slice CT. The scan coverage of 4-dimensional CT for radiation therapy is typically the whole lung, while the coverage for average CT should be limited for the tumor or the heart region for diagnosis. Radiation dose for 4-dimensional CT is about 50 mGy, and should be less than 5 mGy for average CT. Two data acquisition modes can be used in 4-dimensional CT: cine CT and low-pitch helical

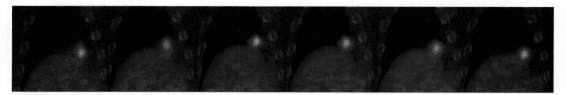

Fig. 12. A 4-dimensional PET/CT patient study. The acquisition time for the 4-dimensional PET scan was 13 minutes, and the PET data were gated into 6 phases. Attenuation of the 4-dimensional PET data was corrected with the corresponding 4-dimensional CT data. Quantification of the tumor in SUV went from 5.0 in the static PET scan without gating to 8.5 in the end-expiration phase of the 4-dimensional PET scan.

CT. Both acquisitions scan the prescribed volume for over 1 breath cycle plus 1 (or 2/3) gantry rotation cycle. Cine CT uses less radiation and generates thinner slices than low-pitch helical CT. Low-pitch helical CT scans are slightly faster than cine CT, because they do not pause between 2 table positions as in cine CT.[88] The cine CT based 4-dimensional CT is available on 4-, 8-, 16-, and 64-slice CT scanners, whereas the low-pitch helical CT-based 4-dimensional CT is only available on newer 16- and 64-slice CT scanners. Four-dimensional CT is a part of 4-dimensional PET/CT if phase-to-phase matching of the attenuation map is desired in 4-dimensional PET imaging.[56,61,68,69] **Fig. 12** illustrates an example of 4-dimensional PET/CT scan of 6 phases over 13 minutes of data acquisition. Quantification of the tumor in SUV changed from 5 in the static PET image without gating to 8.5 at the end-expiration phase in this example. Model-based image reconstruction can also be applied to 4-dimensional PET,[86] based on the tumor motion from 4-dimensional CT, to deform/register the multiple phases of PET data to a single motion freeze PET data set to reduce the noise in 4-dimensional PET data and to improve PET quantification.[89]

SUMMARY

There has been a tremendous effort in improving both PET/CT and 4-dimensional PET/CT imaging in the last decade. With the development of 4-dimensional CT, the difficulties in imaging the tumor motion with CT in the thorax or the abdomen have been largely eliminated. List-mode data acquisition, although not a new concept, has been very useful in making the workflow of postprocessing the 4-dimensional PET data easier than before. Average CT derived from averaging the high temporal resolution CT images acquired over a respiratory cycle has been shown to be effective in improving the registration of the CT and the PET data, resulting in improvement on quantification of the PET data both for tumor imaging and cardiac imaging. Radiation dose of average CT can be reduced to less than 1 mSv, and application of average CT can be limited to only patients whose PET data and CT data do not register. Four-dimensional PET and 4-dimensional PET/CT are emerging as the next frontier for researchers and clinicians to put into clinical use. The bottleneck in 4-dimensional PET and 4-dimensional PET/CT is the long acquisition time for acquiring the 4-dimensional PET data. It is hoped that future instrumentation can improve the sensitivity of PET imaging so that every whole-body PET scan can become

a 4-dimensional PET scan without any significant increase of the scan time.

REFERENCES

1. Beyer T, Townsend DW, Brun T, et al. A combined PET/CT scanner for clinical oncology. J Nucl Med 2000;41(8):1369–79.
2. Townsend DW, Beyer T. A combined PET/CT scanner: the path to true image fusion. Br J Radiol 2002;75:S24–30.
3. Hutton BF, Braun M. Software for image registration: algorithms, accuracy, efficacy. Semin Nucl Med 2003;33(3):180–92.
4. Slomka P, Baum R. Multimodality image registration with software: state-of-the-art. Eur J Nucl Med Mol Imaging 2009;36(Suppl 1):44–55.
5. Reinartz P, Wieres FJ, Schneider W, et al. Side-by-side reading of PET and CT scans in oncology: which patients might profit from integrated PET/CT? Eur J Nucl Med Mol Imaging 2004;31(11):1456–61.
6. Wahl RL. Why nearly all PET of abdominal and pelvic cancers will be performed as PET/CT. J Nucl Med 2004;45:82S–95S.
7. Goerres GW, von Schulthess GK, Steinert HC. Why most PET of lung and head-and-neck cancer will be PET/CT. J Nucl Med 2004;45(Suppl 1):66S–71S.
8. Mawlawi O, Townsend DW. Multimodality imaging: an update on PET/CT technology. Eur J Nucl Med Mol Imagin 2009;36(Suppl 1):S15–29.
9. Hricak H, Choi BI, Scott AM, et al. Global trends in hybrid imaging. Radiology 2010;257(2):498–506.
10. Blodgett TM, Meltzer CC, Townsend DW. PET/CT: form and function. Radiology 2007;242(2):360–85.
11. Rohren EM, Turkington TG, Coleman RE. Clinical applications of PET in oncology. Radiology 2004;231(2):305–32.
12. Bradley J, Thorstad WL, Mutic S, et al. Impact of FDG-PET on radiation therapy volume delineation in non-small-cell lung cancer. Int J Radiat Oncol Biol Phys 2004;59(1):78–86.
13. Ciernik IF, Dizendorf E, Baumert BG, et al. Radiation treatment planning with an integrated positron emission and computer tomography (PET/CT): a feasibility study. Int J Radiat Oncol Biol Phys 2003;57(3):853–63.
14. Mah K, Caldwell CB, Ung YC, et al. The impact of (18)FDG-PET on target and critical organs in CT-based treatment planning of patients with poorly defined non-small-cell lung carcinoma: a prospective study. Int J Radiat Oncol Biol Phys 2002;52(2):339–50.
15. van Baardwijk A, Baumert BG, Bosmans G, et al. The current status of FDG-PET in tumour volume definition in radiotherapy treatment planning. Cancer Treat Rev 2006;32(4):245–60.

16. Messa C, Di Muzio N, Picchio M, et al. PET/CT and radiotherapy. Q J Nucl Med Mol Imaging 2006;50(1): 4–14.

17. Di Carli MF, Dorbala S, Meserve J, et al. Clinical myocardial perfusion PET/CT. J Nucl Med 2007; 48(5):783–93.

18. Stewart RD, Li XA. BGRT: biologically guided radiation therapy - the future is fast approaching. Med Phys 2007;34(10):3739–51.

19. Zaidi H, Pan T. Recent advances in hybrid imaging for radiation therapy planning: the cutting edge. PET Clinics 2011;6(2):207–26.

20. Weber WA. Monitoring tumor response to therapy with 18F-FLT PET. J Nucl Med 2010;51(6):841–4.

21. Gregory DL, Hicks RJ, Hogg A, et al. Effect of PET/CT on management of patients with non-small cell lung cancer: results of a prospective study with 5-year survival data. J Nucl Med 2012;53(7):1007–15.

22. Zaidi H, Vees H, Wissmeyer M. Molecular PET/CT imaging-guided radiation therapy treatment planning. Acad Radiol 2009;16(9):1108–33.

23. Steenbakkers RJ, Duppen JC, Fitton I, et al. Reduction of observer variation using matched CT-PET for lung cancer delineation: a three-dimensional analysis. Int J Radiat Oncol Biol Phys 2006;64(2): 435–48.

24. Ashamalla H, Rafla S, Parikh K, et al. The contribution of integrated PET/CT to the evolving definition of treatment volumes in radiation treatment planning in lung cancer. Int J Radiat Oncol Biol Phys 2005; 63(4):1016–23.

25. Erdi YE, Rosenzweig K, Erdi AK, et al. Radiotherapy treatment planning for patients with non-small cell lung cancer using positron emission tomography (PET). Radiother Oncol 2002;62(1):51–60.

26. Schwartz DL, Ford EC, Rajendran J, et al. FDG-PET/CT-guided intensity modulated head and neck radiotherapy: a pilot investigation. Head Neck 2005;27(6):478–87.

27. Valliant JF. A bridge not too far: linking disciplines through molecular imaging probes. J Nucl Med 2010;51(8):1258–68.

28. Chao KS, Bosch WR, Mutic S, et al. A novel approach to overcome hypoxic tumor resistance: Cu-ATSM-guided intensity-modulated radiation therapy. Int J Radiat Oncol Biol Phys 2001;49(4): 1171–82.

29. Kinahan PE, Hasegawa BH, Beyer T. X-ray-based attenuation correction for positron emission tomography/computed tomography scanners. Semin Nucl Med 2003;33(3):166–79.

30. Zaidi H, Hasegawa BH. Determination of the attenuation map in emission tomography. J Nucl Med 2003;44(2):291–315.

31. Zaidi H, Montandon ML, Alavi A. Advances in attenuation correction techniques in PET. PET Clinics 2007;2(2):191–217.

32. Zasadny KR, Wahl RL. Standardized uptake values of normal tissues at PET with 2-[fluorine-18]-fluoro-2-deoxy-D-glucose: variations with body weight and a method for correction. Radiology 1993; 189(3):847–50.

33. Keyes JW Jr. SUV: standard uptake or silly useless value? J Nucl Med 1995;36(10):1836–9.

34. Basu S, Zaidi H, Houseni M, et al. Novel quantitative techniques for assessing regional and global function and structure based on modern imaging modalities: implications for normal variation, aging and diseased states. Semin Nucl Med 2007;37(3): 223–39.

35. Antoch G, Freudenberg LS, Egelhof T, et al. Focal tracer uptake: a potential artifact in contrast-enhanced dual-modality PET/CT scans. J Nucl Med 2002;43(10):1339–42.

36. Vogel WV, van Dalen JA, Wiering B, et al. Evaluation of image registration in PET/CT of the liver and recommendations for optimized imaging. J Nucl Med 2007;48(6):910–9.

37. Osman MM, Cohade C, Nakamoto Y, et al. Respiratory motion artifacts on PET emission images obtained using CT attenuation correction on PET-CT. Eur J Nucl Med Mol Imaging 2003;30(4):603–6.

38. Osman MM, Cohade C, Nakamoto Y, et al. Clinically significant inaccurate localization of lesions with PET/CT: frequency in 300 patients. J Nucl Med 2003;44(2):240–3.

39. Goerres GW, Kamel E, Seifert B, et al. Accuracy of image coregistration of pulmonary lesions in patients with non-small cell lung cancer using an integrated PET/CT system. J Nucl Med 2002;43(11):1469–75.

40. Beyer T, Antoch G, Muller S, et al. Acquisition protocol considerations for combined PET/CT imaging. J Nucl Med 2004;45(Suppl 1):25S–35S.

41. Beyer T, Rosenbaum S, Veit P, et al. Respiration artifacts in whole-body (18)F-FDG PET/CT studies with combined PET/CT tomographs employing spiral CT technology with 1 to 16 detector rows. Eur J Nucl Med Mol Imaging 2005;32(12):1429–39.

42. Pan T, Mawlawi O, Nehmeh SA, et al. Attenuation correction of PET images with respiration-averaged CT images in PET/CT. J Nucl Med 2005;46(9):1481–7.

43. Chi PC, Mawlawi O, Luo D, et al. Effects of respiration-averaged computed tomography on positron emission tomography/computed tomography quantification and its potential impact on gross tumor volume delineation. Int J Radiat Oncol Biol Phys 2008;71(3):890–9.

44. Kawano T, Ohtake E, Inoue T. Deep-inspiration breath-hold PET/CT of lung cancer: maximum standardized uptake value analysis of 108 patients. J Nucl Med 2008;49(8):1223–31.

45. Gould KL, Pan T, Loghin C, et al. Frequent diagnostic errors in cardiac PET/CT due to misregistration of CT attenuation and emission PET images: a definitive

analysis of causes, consequences, and corrections. J Nucl Med 2007;48(7):1112–21.

46. Young H, Baum R, Cremerius U, et al. Measurement of clinical and subclinical tumour response using [18F]-fluorodeoxyglucose and positron emission tomography: review and 1999 EORTC recommendations. European Organization for Research and Treatment of Cancer (EORTC) PET Study Group. Eur J Cancer 1999;35(13):1773–82.

47. Goerres GW, Burger C, Schwitter MR, et al. PET/CT of the abdomen: optimizing the patient breathing pattern. Eur Radiol 2003;13(4):734–9.

48. Fitton I, Steenbakkers RJ, Zijp L, et al. Retrospective attenuation correction of PET data for radiotherapy planning using a free breathing CT. Radiother Oncol 2007;83(1):42–8.

49. Gilman MD, Fischman AJ, Krishnasetty V, et al. Optimal CT breathing protocol for combined thoracic PET/CT. AJR Am J Roentgenol 2006;187(5):1357–60.

50. Nye JA, Esteves F, Votaw JR. Minimizing artifacts resulting from respiratory and cardiac motion by optimization of the transmission scan in cardiac PET/CT. Med Phys 2007;34(6):1901–6.

51. Pan T, Mawlawi O, Luo D, et al. Attenuation correction of PET cardiac data with low-dose average CT in PET/CT. Med Phys 2006;33(10):3931–8.

52. Chi PC, Mawlawi O, Nehmeh SA, et al. Design of respiration averaged CT for attenuation correction of the PET data from PET/CT. Med Phys 2007; 34(6):2039–47.

53. Cook RA, Carnes G, Lee TY, et al. Respiration-averaged CT for attenuation correction in canine cardiac PET/CT. J Nucl Med 2007;48(5):811–8.

54. Huang TC, Mok GS, Wang SJ, et al. Attenuation correction of PET images with interpolated average CT for thoracic tumors. Phys Med Biol 2011;56(8): 2559–67.

55. Wu TH, Zhang G, Wang SJ, et al. Low-dose interpolated average CT for attenuation correction in cardiac PET/CT. Nucl Instrum Meth A 2010;619(1–3):361–4.

56. Nagel CC, Bosmans G, Dekker AL, et al. Phased attenuation correction in respiration correlated computed tomography/positron emitted tomography. Med Phys 2006;33(6):1840–7.

57. Wells RG, Ruddy TD, DeKemp RA, et al. Single-phase CT aligned to gated PET for respiratory motion correction in cardiac PET/CT. J Nucl Med 2010;51(8):1182–90.

58. Ponisch F, Richter C, Just U, et al. Attenuation correction of four dimensional (4D) PET using phase-correlated 4D-computed tomography. Phys Med Biol 2008;53(13):N259–68.

59. Alessio AM, Kohlmyer S, Branch K, et al. Cine CT for attenuation correction in cardiac PET/CT. J Nucl Med 2007;48(5):794–801.

60. Nehmeh SA, Erdi YE, Rosenzweig KE, et al. Reduction of respiratory motion artifacts in PET imaging of lung cancer by respiratory correlated dynamic PET: methodology and comparison with respiratory gated PET. J Nucl Med 2003;44(10):1644–8.

61. Erdi YE, Nehmeh SA, Pan T, et al. The CT motion quantitation of lung lesions and its impact on PET-measured SUVs. J Nucl Med 2004;45(8):1287–92.

62. Mageras GS, Pevsner A, Yorke ED, et al. Measurement of lung tumor motion using respiration-correlated CT. Int J Radiat Oncol Biol Phys 2004; 60(3):933–41.

63. Nehmeh SA, Erdi YE, Meirelles GS, et al. Deep-inspiration breath-hold PET/CT of the thorax. J Nucl Med 2007;48(1):22–6.

64. Meirelles GS, Erdi YE, Nehmeh SA, et al. Deep-inspiration breath-hold PET/CT: clinical findings with a new technique for detection and characterization of thoracic lesions. J Nucl Med 2007;48(5):712–9.

65. Torizuka T, Tanizaki Y, Kanno T, et al. Single 20-second acquisition of deep-inspiration breath-hold PET/CT: clinical feasibility for lung cancer. J Nucl Med 2009;50(10):1579–84.

66. Nehmeh SA, Erdi YE, Ling CC, et al. Effect of respiratory gating on reducing lung motion artifacts in PET imaging of lung cancer. Med Phys 2002;29(3): 366–71.

67. Nehmeh SA, Erdi YE, Ling CC, et al. Effect of respiratory gating on quantifying PET images of lung cancer. J Nucl Med 2002;43(7):876–81.

68. Nehmeh SA, Erdi YE, Pan T, et al. Four-dimensional (4D) PET/CT imaging of the thorax. Med Phys 2004; 31(12):3179–86.

69. Nehmeh SA, Erdi YE, Pan T, et al. Quantitation of respiratory motion during 4D-PET/CT acquisition. Med Phys 2004;31(6):1333–8.

70. Boucher L, Rodrigue S, Lecomte R, et al. Respiratory gating for 3-dimensional PET of the thorax: feasibility and initial results. J Nucl Med 2004;45(2):214–9.

71. Pevsner A, Nehmeh SA, Humm JL, et al. Effect of motion on tracer activity determination in CT attenuation corrected PET images: a lung phantom study. Med Phys 2005;32(7):2358–62.

72. Martinez-Möller A, Zikic D, Botnar R, et al. Dual cardiac respiratory gated PET: implementation and results from a feasibility study. Eur J Nucl Med Mol Imaging 2007;34(9):1447–54.

73. Klein GJ, Reutter BW, Ho MH, et al. Real-time system for respiratory-cardiac gating in positron tomography. IEEE Trans Nucl Sci 1998;45(4):2139–43.

74. Visvikis D, Lamare F, Bruyant P, et al. Respiratory motion in positron emission tomography for oncology applications: problems and solutions. Nucl Instr Meth A 2006;569(2):453–7.

75. Rahmim A, Rousset O, Zaidi H. Strategies for motion tracking and correction in PET. PET Clinics 2007; 2(2):251–66.

76. Keall PJ, Mageras GS, Balter JM, et al. The management of respiratory motion in radiation oncology

report of AAPM Task Group 76. Med Phys 2006; 33(10):3874–900.

77. Low DA, Nystrom M, Kalinin E, et al. A method for the reconstruction of four-dimensional synchronized CT scans acquired during free breathing. Med Phys 2003;30(6):1254–63.

78. Pan T, Lee TY, Rietzel E, et al. 4D-CT imaging of a volume influenced by respiratory motion on multi-slice CT. Med Phys 2004;31(2):333–40.

79. Keall PJ, Starkschall G, Shukla H, et al. Acquiring 4D thoracic CT scans using a multislice helical method. Phys Med Biol 2004;49(10):2053–67.

80. Pan T, Sun X, Luo D. Improvement of the cine-CT based 4D-CT imaging. Med Phys 2007;34(11): 4499–503.

81. Papathanassiou D, Becker S, Amir R, et al. Respiratory motion artifact in the liver dome on FDG PET/CT: comparison of attenuation correction with CT and a caesium external source. Eur J Nucl Med Mol Imaging 2005;32(12):1422–8.

82. Wu TH, Huang YH, Lee JJ, et al. Radiation exposure during transmission measurements: comparison between CT- and germanium-based techniques with a current PET scanner. Eur J Nucl Med Mol Imaging 2004;31(1):38–43.

83. Riegel AC, Ahmad M, Sun X, et al. Dose calculation with respiration-averaged CT processed from cine CT without a respiratory surrogate. Med Phys 2008;35(12):5738–47.

84. Hoffman EJ, Phelps ME, Wisenberg G, et al. Electrocardiographic gating in positron emission computed tomography. J Comput Assist Tomogr 1979;3(6): 733–9.

85. Vedam SS, Keall PJ, Kini VR, et al. Acquiring a four-dimensional computed tomography dataset using an external respiratory signal. Phys Med Biol 2003; 48(1):45–62.

86. Rahmim A, Tang J, Zaidi H. Four-dimensional (4D) image reconstruction strategies in dynamic PET: beyond conventional independent frame reconstruction. Med Phys 2009;36(8):3654–70.

87. Kinahan PE, Vesselle H, MacDonald L, et al. Whole-body respiratory gated PET/CT. J Nucl Med 2006; 47(1):187P.

88. Pan T. Comparison of helical and cine acquisitions for 4D-CT imaging with multislice CT. Med Phys 2005;32(2):627–34.

89. Li T, Thorndyke B, Schreibmann E, et al. Model-based image reconstruction for four-dimensional PET. Med Phys 2006;33(5):1288–98.

Four-Dimensional Image Reconstruction Strategies in Cardiac-Gated and Respiratory-Gated PET Imaging

Arman Rahmim, PhD[a],*, Jing Tang, PhD[b],
Habib Zaidi, PhD, PD[c,d,e]

KEYWORDS

- PET • Motion tracking • Motion correction • Cardiac gating • Respiratory gating
- 4D image reconstruction • 5D image reconstruction

KEY POINTS

- Cardiac and/or respiratory gating leads to enhanced noise levels, thus producing images with reduced quality.
- Direct four-dimensional (4D) PET image reconstruction incorporating motion compensation provides a very promising alternative to this problem.
- A wide-ranging choice of techniques are available in research settings but have not yet been used in the clinic.
- The development of advanced 4D physical anthropomorphic phantoms and computational models will benefit research in cardiac-gated and respiratory-gated PET imaging.

INTRODUCTION

Positron emission tomography (PET) is a powerful modality for numerous oncologic and cardiac imaging applications. However, when PET is used for chest or upper abdomen examinations, respiratory motion can lead to blurring and distortion of the images. Cardiac imaging applications also suffer from both cardiac and respiratory movements of the heart. Much worthwhile research has focused during the last decade on developing motion compensation techniques to provide more accurate PET images[1,2]; e.g. for the diagnosis and assessment of lung and upper abdomen cancer. It is expected that better PET images will lead to improved detection of small lesions and enhance the ability to assess the extent of the cancer. In some cases, more accurate assessment of chest and upper abdomen lesions may mean that patients can avoid the trauma and expense of surgery. It is expected that physicians will be able to make more informed decisions about how to treat patients with cancer

This work was supported by the Swiss National Science Foundation under grant SNSF 31003A-135576, Geneva Cancer League, the National Science Foundation under grant ECCS 1228091 and the Indo-Swiss Joint Research Programme ISJRP 138866.

[a] Division of Nuclear Medicine, Department of Radiology, Johns Hopkins University, Johns Hopkins Outpatient Centre, Room 3245, 601 N. Caroline Street, Baltimore, MD 21287, USA; [b] Department of Electrical & Computer Engineering, Oakland University, 2200 N Squirrel Road, Rochester, MI 48309, USA; [c] Division of Nuclear Medicine and Molecular Imaging, Geneva University Hospital, Geneva CH-1211, Switzerland; [d] Geneva Neuroscience Center, Geneva University, Geneva CH-1211, Switzerland; [e] Department of Nuclear Medicine and Molecular Imaging, University Medical Center Groningen, University of Groningen, Groningen 9700 RB, Netherlands

* Corresponding author.
E-mail address: arahmim1@jhmi.edu

PET Clin 8 (2013) 51–67
http://dx.doi.org/10.1016/j.cpet.2012.10.005

lesions in the chest and upper abdomen, particularly when enhanced PET imaging is used in conjunction with structural (CT or MR) scanning. Similarly, in cardiac imaging applications, enhanced clinical tasks will be possible, as elaborated shortly.

A solution to the problem of motion is to perform cardiac and/or respiratory gating of the data, followed by reconstructions of individual gated datasets. However, gating leads to enhanced noise levels and images of reduced quality are generated, which in turn can also lead to enhanced noise-induced bias and variance in kinetic parameters.[1]

An advanced approach to PET imaging is to move beyond pure gating and to obtain enhanced images by making collective use of the gated data sets. Two general schemes may be considered: (1) postreconstruction registration and summation of the independently reconstructed images (eg,[3–7]); (2) incorporation of motion information within the reconstruction algorithm: this latter approach is broadly referred to as four-dimensional (4D) reconstruction, which is the topic reviewed in this article. Asma and colleagues[8] and Chun and Fessler[9] theoretically analyzed and compared postreconstruction versus 4D reconstruction approaches with motion compensation, and showed that noise variance in the latter is less than or comparable with the variance in the former, and the gap between them is larger when less regularization is used[8] and when the gate frames have significantly different counts.[9]

Dynamic imaging and motion-compensated imaging methods overlap in the sense that they both deal with varying activity distributions over time, and 4D methods have been developed for both. The underlying bases of the two are different and need to be distinguished from one another. In particular, some types of motion (and thus certain changes in voxel intensity) are physically/anatomically impossible. 4D image reconstruction algorithms applicable to dynamic imaging have been reviewed elsewhere,[10] whereas here we focus on techniques to model and incorporate motion. Overall, we believe that strategies attempting to apply general 4D PET image reconstruction techniques (such as use of temporal basis functions) to motion compensation (eg, Refs.[11,12]) remain to be further refined or constrained to ensure meaningful reconstructions. Aiming to exploit the periodic nature of cardiac motion, a promising approach[13] was to use temporal Fourier harmonic basis functions to model voxel intensity variation across the gates.

The first section of this article reviews application of 4D image reconstruction methods to cardiac imaging applications, which may involve cardiac or respiratory gating. The next section reviews applications beyond cardiac imaging (particularly, oncology) involving respiratory motion correction only. Some important areas of future research are discussed at the end.

CARDIAC IMAGING APPLICATIONS

Cardiac movements introduce notable visual and quantitative degradations in PET imaging: the base of the heart typically moves 9 to 14 mm toward the apex, and the myocardial walls thicken from approximately 10 mm to more than 15 mm between the end-diastole and end-systole.[14] The motivation behind motion correction in cardiac imaging is two-fold:

i. To further improve the quality of cardiac PET images (noise, resolution) so as to enhance identifiability of radiotracer uptake defects in the left ventricle (LV) by clinicians, because regions of decreased radiotracer uptake can indicate hibernating or infracted myocardial tissue.[15] This finding is also important when applying quantitative measures of perfusion and metabolic parameters in dynamic compartmental modeling studies.[16]

ii. Measurement of motion itself can be useful for characterizing cardiac function.[17] Measures such as ejection fraction and regional wall thickening may be derived from a measure of contractile motion in this way.

We first focus on efforts using cardiac gating only (additional respiratory gating in the context of cardiac imaging is discussed later). Postreconstruction motion correction approaches involving nonrigid registration and summation of individually gated cardiac images have been reviewed elsewhere.[1,2,18]

Cardiac Motion Estimation Methods

Cardiac motion (ie, the contraction of LV during the cardiac cycle) was commonly described by relatively global measures before techniques were developed to estimate the dense motion vector fields (ie, voxel-by-voxel point correspondences). Global parameters such as ejection fraction,[19] longitudinal shortening,[20] radial contraction, and wall thickening[21] provide diagnostic information about the cardiac function. Other than providing a more elaborate description of cardiac motion, a major objective of obtaining the dense motion field is to compensate for motion in cardiac-gated imaging and arrive at reduced blurring artifacts without intensifying noise levels.[22–25]

Compared with emission tomography imaging, tagged MR imaging provides a more favorable environment for calculation of the dense motion field (myocardial tagging involves production of a spatial pattern of saturated magnetization, eg, at end-diastole, and then imaging the resulting deformation of the pattern as the heart contracts through the cardiac cycle).[26–28] The difference in intensities between tagged and untagged regions allows tracking of the motion of underlying tissues. Young and colleagues[29] presented a method for tracking stripe motion in the image plane and showed how the information could be incorporated into a finite-element model of underlying deformation. The method provided a framework to combine high-level global constraints (eg, smoothness and connectivity) with low-level local constraints (eg, dark, linear features). Park and colleagues[30] presented a technique using a class of physics-based deformable models allowing parameterized deformations that captured the motion of the LV. Ozturk and McVeigh[31] used 4D B-splines to interpolate the motion between the tracked myocardial points. The 4D displacement field formed by combining the two-dimensional (2D) fields, as derived from the short-axis and long-axis image planes, could be used to track the deformation of points anywhere within the myocardium. Osman and colleagues[32] proposed a method that estimates cardiac motion applied to spatial modulation of magnetization (SPAMM)-tagged MR images. The SPAMM-tagged images have a collection of distinct spectral peaks in the Fourier domain, each of which contains information about the motion in a certain direction. The inverse Fourier transform of just one of these peaks is a complex image, the phase of which is linearly related to a directional component of the true motion. These investigators defined the harmonic phase (HARP) image to be the principle value of the phase of the complex image and used the HARP image to measure small displacement fields. The main characteristic of this method is its computational simplicity.

We discuss these methods for tagged MR images not only for the completeness of the literature review on cardiac motion estimation but also to resonate with the recent emergence of integrated PET/MR scanners.[33,34] Recent work by Petibon and colleagues[35] applied cardiac wall motion estimated from tagged MR images in PET image reconstruction for simultaneous PET/MR. This preliminary work reported improved perfusion defect detection using a physical phantom.

For other imaging modalities, different extensions of the classic optical flow approach of Horn and Schunck[36] have been commonly applied.

The optical flow technique assumes that a moving point in a sequence of images does not change its intensity. The classic approach invokes local Taylor series approximations [using partial derivatives with respect to the spatial and temporal coordinates]. It was first applied directly to 2D cardiac images in Refs.[37,38] Because 2D motion is inadequate to describe cardiac motion vectors, three-dimensional (3D) extension of the algorithm was provided by Song and Leahy[39] and Zhou and colleagues[40] on CT cardiac sequences. Klein and colleagues[3,9] used a nonuniform elastic regularization function inspired from a linear elastic material model.[41] The motion field is regularized by an energy function constraining the source volume as if it were a physical elastic material being deformed by external forces. In several works in which simultaneous gated image reconstruction and motion estimation were performed,[25,30,42] algorithms including similar regularization via the strain energy function were implemented for the purpose of myocardium motion estimation. These works reported improved noise and resolution characteristics in the reconstructed images (**Fig. 1**). In addition, Gravier and colleagues[24] also performed cardiac motion estimation via the optical flow method, which they subsequently incorporated as temporal regularization in 4D image reconstruction, showing improved accuracy of cardiac images without causing any significant cross-frame blurring.

Optical flow techniques assume that a moving point in a sequence of images does not change its intensity. This assumption may be violated in emission tomography because of the limited spatial resolution (and the resulting partial volume effect), particularly as the myocardium expands and becomes thin in the end-diastolic phase. An alternative is to invoke the continuity equation describing conservation of mass (here, intensity), resulting in an additional term relative to classic optical flow (and sometimes referred to as extended optical flow)[39]; such an approach was recently used by Dawood and colleagues[43] for cardiac motion estimation.

Optical flow algorithms are known for the aperture problem wherein there is not enough information in a small area to uniquely determine motion perpendicular to the direction of the local gradient of the image intensity.[44,45] This problem is commonly tackled via introduction of additional constraints. Nonetheless, the true motion cannot be recovered without a priori knowledge of the motion. Klein and colleagues[9] performed qualitative analysis on tracking the cardiac twist in the healthy PET myocardium. The motion field estimated from PET images, cine MR images, and

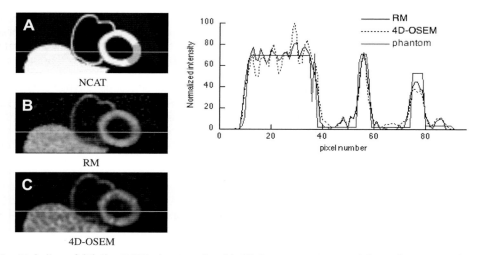

Fig. 1. Sagittal slice of (A) the NCAT phantom (truth), (B) image reconstructed from the proposed integrated image reconstruction and motion (RM) estimation algorithm, and (C) image reconstructed using the conventional OSEM (ordered subset expectation–maximization) algorithm plus 4D postreconstruction filtering. Profiles of the images along the section indicated by the line. (*Reprinted from* Mair BA, Gilland DR, Sun J. Estimation of images and nonrigid deformations in gated emission CT. IEEE Trans Med Imaging 2006;25(9):1140; with permission.)

tagged MR images was compared. The conclusion was that the component of motion normal to the ventricular surfaces could be accurately estimated; however, because of uniformity in the healthy myocardium in PET imaging, the torsion component was considerably more difficult to track. Cine MR images with higher resolution did not augment the ability of the optical flow technique in terms of catching the twist motion. Only tagged MR images had sufficient features for the algorithm to accurately estimate the motion.

The performance of the optical flow technique to estimate cardiac motion from emission tomography images was evaluated quantitatively by Tang and colleagues.[46] Using the 4D NCAT (NURBs (nonuniform rational B-splines) Cardiac Torso) phantom with a known motion vector field, the study confirmed that the optical flow technique could not appropriately estimate tangential motion for uniform myocardial perfusion patterns. It also showed that without detection of the tangential motion, the estimated radial motion also deviates from the truth, because the motion components are correlated with each other.

Besides optical flow methods, some other techniques were investigated for motion-compensated image reconstruction. For example, the motion-frozen technique by Slomka and colleagues,[47] originally applied to single-photon emission CT (SPECT), involved detecting the epicardial and endocardial surfaces and tracking their movements, followed by extrapolation of the movements

of the surfaces to other points. The technique was also applied in PET image reconstruction,[8] resulting in significantly enhanced (*P*<.05) contrast and contrast/noise ratios in fluorodeoxyglucose myocardial viability images.

Reconstruction Methods

In the following sections, four general 4D reconstruction approaches are reviewed: those in which motion estimation is performed (1–3) before or (4) during 4D image reconstruction.

1. Interiterative temporal smoothing: given the estimated motion vectors enabling tracking of any given voxel across the cardiac gates, this approach imposes temporal smoothing across the gated images after every iteration of the reconstruction algorithm. Such an approach was suggested by Brankov and colleagues,[48] who in addition replaced the uniform-voxel framework with mesh modeling within image reconstruction[49] (an efficient image description based on nonuniform sampling; mesh nodes are placed more densely in image regions having finer detail). However, the investigators seem to have abandoned this approach in favor of postreconstruction motion-compensated filtering in later publications.[50,51] Overall, spatial[52,53] or temporal[54,55] interiteration filtering methods are ad hoc (eg, are not proved to be convergent). A more theoretically sound and more popular approach is discussed next.

2. Bayesian maximum a posteriori (MAP) reconstruction: MAP methods[56] attempt to address the ill-posed nature of emission tomography reconstruction via inclusion of spatial or temporal priors.[57] Instead of seeking an image estimate $\vec{f}$ that maximizes the Poisson log-likelihood function $L(\vec{f})$ as is the case with the regular expectation-maximization (EM) algorithm,[58,59] MAP methods seek to maximize the MAP function $L(\vec{f}) - \beta V(\vec{f})$, where $V(\vec{f})$ is a potential function that regularizes the objective function (commonly by penalizing intensity variations within spatial neighborhoods), and β is the MAP hyperparameter to be set by the user for the particular imaging task. A common (although approximate) iterative solution to the MAP formulation can be reached via the one-step-late (OSL) approach of Green,[60] arriving at

$$\vec{f}^{new} = \frac{\vec{f}^{old}}{P^T \vec{1} + \beta \left.\dfrac{\partial V(\vec{f})}{\partial \vec{f}}\right|_{\vec{f} = \vec{f}^{old}}} P^T \frac{\vec{y}}{P \vec{f}^{old}} \qquad (1)$$

where $\vec{f}^{old}$ and $\vec{f}^{new}$ denote the previous and updated image estimates, $\vec{y}$ is the projection space data, P is the system matrix modeling the probabilities of detection, and $\vec{1}$ is a column vector with all elements equal to 1.

In addition, Gravier and Yang[61] used a MAP formulation to encourage smoothing across the gated frames, given knowledge of voxel movements from the estimated motion vector field. As an example, denoting the estimated activity for a given gate q (q = 1…Q) as $\vec{f}_q$, the following penalty V_t was considered:

$$V_t = \sum_{q=1}^{Q} \sum_{j=1}^{J} \left[[\vec{f}_q]_j - \frac{1}{Q-1} \sum_{\substack{p=1 \\ p \neq q}}^{Q} [M_{p \to q} \vec{f}_p]_j \right]^2 \qquad (2)$$

where the subscript j denotes the particular voxel (j = 1…J) in the image, and $M_{p \to q}$ denotes the estimated motion matrix transforming a given image $\vec{f}_q$ to its corresponding distribution in gate p given the estimate motion vectors. The investigators introduced a generalized weighted formulation[24,62] to this expression to weight intergate variations in voxel intensities depending on gate separation (higher weights for nearer gates).

A similar approach was taken by Lalush and colleagues[63,64] but the motion was assumed to be known a priori. However, they obtained

similar results when no motion information was considered (ie, $M_{p \to q}$ was set to the identity matrix). This result may have been caused by the limited resolution of their scanner, but has been pursued similarly in several subsequent works.[65–68]

3. The MAP-OSL algorithm (1) of Green[60] is based on an approximation (and breaks down for large values of β). In addition, it is a nontrivial task to select the parameters associated with the prior/penalty term (which play an important role in the image quality) and this is often achieved through trial-and-error. These methods treat the same moving object as different temporal reconstructions that are merely temporally correlated. Nevertheless, a more concrete approach would involve a truly 4D approach, in which the estimated deformations are incorporated within a unified cost function to be optimized (for a single object). Such an approach was proposed and investigated by Qiao and colleagues,[69] Li and colleagues,[70] and Lamare and colleagues,[71] although originally for respiratory gating applications but later also used for cardiac gating.[72] In this approach, the measured nonrigid motion (estimated from the gated images) is modeled in the image-space component of the system matrix of the EM algorithm, and a truly 4D EM reconstruction algorithm has been achieved. This approach is promising because of its accurate and comprehensive modeling of the relation of a moving object to detected events. Introducing a time/gate-varying system matrix P, including decomposition[73–75] into the geometric component G, diagonal normalization N and attenuation A matrices, as well as $M_{1 \to q}$ modeling the motion transformation from the reference gate 1 to existing frame q ($P = NAGM_{1 \to q}$), one arrives at the 4D EM update algorithm to estimate the image at the reference gate:

$$\vec{f}^{new} = \frac{\vec{f}^{old}}{\vec{s}} \sum_{q=1}^{Q} M_{1 \to q}^T G^T \frac{\vec{Y}_q}{GM_{1 \to q} \vec{f}^{old}} \qquad (3)$$

where the sensitivity image $\vec{s}$ is given by

$$\vec{s} = \sum_{q=1}^{Q} M_{1 \to q}^T G^T A^T N^T \vec{1} \qquad (4)$$

This approach is analogous to motion-corrected EM reconstructions in brain imaging that move beyond purely correcting[76–78] individual events for motion and that result in modified sensitivity images to account for the impact of motion on probabilities of detection.[79–83]

4. Commonly in the literature, cardiac motion is estimated after reconstruction of individual gated frames; and in the techniques outlined earlier, the extracted motion information is used in subsequent 4D reconstructions to yield enhanced images. However, Gilland and colleagues[22,23,42] hypothesized that, given the close link between the image reconstruction and motion estimation steps, a simultaneous method of estimating the two is better able to (1) reduce motion blur and compensate for poor signal-to-noise (SNR) ratios and to (2) improve the accuracy of the estimated motion. Their proposed algorithm worked by 2-step minimization of a joint energy functional term (which included both image likelihood and motion-matching terms). This work was also extended from a 2-frame approach to the complete cardiac cycle by Gilland and colleagues.[84]

The approach taken by Jacobson and Fessler[85,86] considered a parametric Poisson model for gated PET measurements involving the activity distribution as unknown as well as a set of deformation parameters describing the motion of the image throughout the scan (from gate to gate). By maximizing the log-likelihood for this model, a technique referred to as joint estimation with deformation modeling was used to determine both the image and deformation parameter estimates jointly from the full set of measured data. A similar motion-aware likelihood function was used by Blume and colleagues,[87] although using a distinct optimization scheme and depicting more convincing results, which is shown in **Fig. 2**. By comparison, the techniques described earlier estimate a single image and $N - 1$ deformations, whereas the method of Gilland and colleagues estimates N images and $N - 1$ motion deformations, thus involving a larger number of unknowns; the cost function it uses does not involve deformations in the log-likelihood term, thus potentially simplifying the optimization task. The aforementioned trade-off remains to be elaborately studied.

Dual-Gated Imaging

Respiratory motion of the heart is comparable with myocardial wall thickness[88] and introduces considerable degradations in quantitative accuracy of images[89] and quality of polar maps.[90] Increasingly more attention has been paid to dual gating of the heart in human and animal studies.[88,91–100] Different hardware gating devices developed in academic and corporate settings were exploited to achieve this goal and are described in the article by Bettinardi and colleagues elsewhere in this issue.

Rigid Versus Nonrigid Modeling of the Respiratory Motion of the Heart

Respiratory motion of the heart has been modeled as rigid within several PET[89,101] and SPECT[102] reconstructions. There exists some evidence to this end: analysis[103] of 20 sets of 4D respiratory-gated

| MC | IG | 4D-a | PRRS | 4D-b | JR | IM | OI |

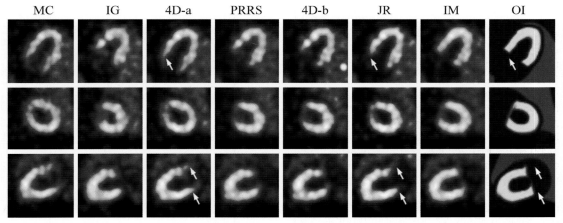

Fig. 2. Selected transverse, coronal, and sagittal slices for different reconstruction scenarios for simulated data (*from left to right*): ML-EM reconstruction of motion-contaminated data (MC), ML-EM reconstruction of the individual gates (IG), 4D method (when motion is estimated from preliminary reconstructions) (*4D-a*), postreconstruction registration and summation (PRRS), 4D method when different gridding is used to estimate motion (*4D-b*), proposed joint reconstruction (JR), and a motion compensating reconstruction based on the ideal motion (IM). For comparison, the original image (OI) is shown in the last column. (*Reprinted from* Blume M, Martinez-Moller A, Keil A, et al. Joint reconstruction of image and motion in gated positron emission tomography. IEEE Trans Med Imaging 2010;29(11):1896; with permission.)

image data from normal and abnormal humans revealed respiratory motion of the heart (as well as liver, stomach, spleen, and kidneys) to involve for the most part rigid translations downward and to the interior as the diaphragm contracts during inspiration. Furthermore, MR scans performed on 15 normal individuals depicted predominantly translational nature of respiratory-induced movements in upper abdominal organs.[104]

Nonetheless, respiratory motion does induce some nonrigid movements in the heart, as it is pushed and pulled by the diaphragm and other connected tissue: for instance, gated CT studies on dogs[105] recorded an average change of 12% in the total end-diastolic heart volume during forced positive pressure inspiration at 15 cm H_2O. Using echocardiography, similar shape changes were found in human individuals.[106] Furthermore, Klein and colleagues[99] performed quantitative measures of respiratory motion of the heart as extracted from 10 respiratory-gated PET studies. Translations between end-inspiration and end-expiration were often greater than 10 mm and ranged from 1 to more than 20 mm (rigid motion). Moreover, the LV showed nonnegligible compression factors. The LV was generally largest at end-inspiration and smallest at end-expiration. Nonrigid motion was close to 10% in several cases, computed as the product of the 3 extension factors along the x, y, and z directions.

The extension factors were largest along the superior/inferior axis ($\sim$5%), which, given the typical 80-mm to 100-mm dimension of the LV along this direction, would result in a heart image that would be 4 to 5 mm too small if motion was assumed simply rigid. Compared with the average 10-mm thickness of the left ventricular wall, this scaling error may therefore be considerable. However, with the ECAT EXACT HR scanner (CTI/Siemens, Knoxville, TN), only small improvements were observed[99] after performing nonrigid motion modeling. It may be concluded that appropriateness of modeling respiratory motion of the heart as rigid versus nonrigid depends on the resolution of the PET scanner. With wider acceptance of reconstruction algorithms incorporating resolution modeling (also referred to as point-spread-function (PSF) modeling),[107–113] and the resulting resolution improvements down to the 2-mm to 3-mm range in clinical scanners, it is expected that nonrigid modeling approaches would serve as more reliable and accurate models of respiratory motion of the heart. Efforts to this end include: (1) use of affine motion models (strictly speaking, an affine model is nonrigid, but in the literature, often it is a class of its own (ie, rigid vs affine vs nonrigid models): this model extends the rigid

motion model (6 parameters of rotation and translation) to also allow 3 scale[71] and 3 skew parameters[99] and (2) use of nonrigid B-spline models.[91]

Reconstruction Methods

Modeling respiratory motion of the heart as rigid, Livieratos and colleagues[101] transformed individual lines of response (LORs) (ie, via translations and rotations) to compensate for respiratory motion, followed by standard reconstructions of individual cardiac-gated datasets. Nonetheless, this approach, although appropriately compensating for normalization given original LOR coordinates, did not compensate for duration of time each LOR spends outside the field-of-view because of motion, which can be compensated via multiplication factors applied to the motion-compensated events[114] or modifying the sensitivity images through the 4D EM formalism of Eqs. 3 and 4. Invoking the latter approach, Rahmim and colleagues[89] and Chen and colleagues[91] performed 4D respiratory motion compensation for each cardiac phase. A simulated example from Ref.[89] is shown in **Fig. 3**, wherein short-axis reconstructed images, for a given cardiac gate, show noisy reconstructions with additional respiratory gating (left), blurred images with no respiratory gating (middle), and improved definition with favorable noise using 4D reconstruction approach. Receiver operating characteristic analysis involving numerical channelized Hotelling observer studies revealed significant improvements ($P<.0001$) for the task of perfusion defect detection using 4D EM respiratory motion compensation.

It is possible to pursue 4D reconstruction methods that incorporate both cardiac and respiratory gating information, as pursued by Blume and colleagues,[87] within a comprehensive dual-gated framework using 24 total gates. Nonetheless, in practice, the common approach has been to use 4D reconstruction methods to compensate for respiratory motion within each cardiac gate, followed by postreconstruction registration and summing of cardiac-gated images.[91,115]

Five-Dimensional Motion-Corrected Image Reconstruction

Dynamic imaging of the heart enables quantification of tracer uptake, providing valuable information about heart function, including the abilities to quantify myocardial blood flow and coronary flow reserve,[116,117] thus providing several powerful applications.[118–124] Nonetheless, this modality has remained primarily limited to research, and

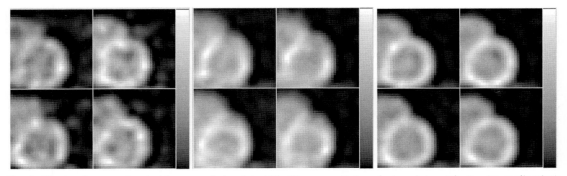

Fig. 3. Short-axis reconstructed images of simulated Rb-82 myocardial perfusion data with 4 noise realizations shown in each set, for the end-diastolic cardiac gate using: *(left)* end-expiration respiratory gate 1, *(middle)* respiratory-nongated data, and *(right)* data processed using 4D EM reconstructions.

remains to be widely adopted in clinical practice; this has been especially related to amplified noise levels caused by subdivision of the data into shorter frames. Novel 4D reconstruction algorithms, aiming to enhance quality and quantitative accuracy of dynamic images, constitute a highly active front and have been reviewed elsewhere.[10,125] Here we discuss some works that have attempted to merge the extra dimensions of cardiac gating and tracer redistribution.

An approach was to use the list-mode capability to first reconstruct the data as gated but static to estimate cardiac motion, followed by application of 4D reconstruction to gated datasets for each dynamic frame.[72] An alternative was to perform 4D image reconstruction to dynamic datasets for each given cardiac gate, followed by postreconstruction filtering across the cardiac gates.[126,127]

By contrast, Jin and colleagues[128] and Gravier and colleagues[62] pursued variations of a more sophisticated five-dimensional (5D) approach of incorporating both dimensions within the reconstruction: they performed preliminary reconstructions to extract the motion vector field; the motion information was then incorporated within objective functions that included weighted variants of (2) penalizing intercardiac-gate intensity variations, although further generalized to also include penalization amongst the dynamic frames. The resulting objective functions were then solved using gradient descent methods. These methods were further refined in Ref.[129] to include a convergent yet fast (ordered subset) reconstruction algorithm framework. Alternatively, Niu and colleagues[130] pursued direct reconstruction of parametric images (from projection data) and incorporated estimated motion vectors within a weighted variant of penalty expression (Eq. 2).

Verhaeghe and colleagues[12] used B-spline temporal basis functions to represent both the temporal and gate dimensions within 5D EM

formulation, resulting in improved noise properties and maintaining sharply defined images (however, see note of caution in introduction regarding treatment of motion in the same sense as dynamic tracer evolution).

A different approach to this problem by Shi and Karl[131,132] involved level set methods wherein a variational framework was developed that collectively incorporated region boundaries (assumed to evolve because of motion) and intensities within them. A coordinate descent algorithm was used alternately minimizing the overall energy function with respect to the boundaries and the intensity values. A downside of this approach is that the intensity is assumed to be constant within the defined regions, although additive noise models were included.

Impact of Mismatched AC

When respiratory gating is not used (ie, emission images are contaminated by respiratory motion), the use of high-speed CT images that capture one phase in the respiratory cycle can lead to AC mismatch, visible artifacts, and notable quantitative degradations.[133,134] Potential solutions to this situation include cine CT, CT mapping (using estimated PET motion vectors, 4D-CT acquisition), and many other approaches. This issue is covered in detail in the article by Pan and Zaidi elsewhere in this issue.

With respiratory gating, as also used in 4D reconstruction methods, application of (1) mismatched or (2) averaged/cine CT for AC can also lead to quantitative degradations,[135] and so forth. Therefore, phase-matching methods seem to be the methods of choice.[136] Unlike respiratory motion, cardiac motion is less important in terms of mismatch between emission and transmission images for AC because the heart sac does not really move with cardiac beating.

BEYOND THE HEART: OTHER IMAGING APPLICATIONS INVOLVING RESPIRATORY MOTION CORRECTION

The 4D methods mentioned in the previous section (for cardiac motion correction) are also applicable to 4D respiratory motion correction. Respiratory motion estimation tasks for different organs are discussed first, as incorporated within 4D reconstruction methods.

Respiratory Motion Estimation Methods

Respiratory motion has been modeled as rigid,[102] affine,[99,137] and nonrigid.[43,138–140] Rigid motion and affine deformation modeling were primarily used in conjunction with event rebinning for the correction of respiratory motion.[71] To rebin the PET data by aligning the LOR of each event to the reference position, the motion can be modeled only as rigid or affine because mapping of an LOR is independent of the event location. Modeling respiratory motion as nonrigid thus requires other motion correction techniques, including incorporating the correction in the image reconstruction process[141] and after reconstruction.[142]

When motion is treated as rigid, it has been quantified by tracking translations of some center of mass along the axial direction[102,143] or in 3D.[144] By contrast, the affine deformation model can be solved using image registration techniques to minimize the least squares difference[99] or mutual information.[137] Nonrigid motion estimation is usually treated as a minimization problem with the cost function consisting of (1) a similarity measure between the image frames and (2) a regularization term on the estimated deformation field. Algorithms differ in the measurement of the image similarity and the selection of the regularization. In the following sections, several representative nonrigid motion estimation algorithms are discussed.

Dawood and colleagues[142] proposed an optical flow-based approach in the process of postreconstruction summation of aligned respiratory gates. The method assumed small motion (for the Taylor expansion) and a locally constant flow (as a means to regularize the problem) per the algorithm developed by Lucas and Kanade (LK).[145] The motion needed to be calculated between adjacent gates (to ensure small motion) rather than between the target gate and successive gates. The LK algorithm is comparatively robust in the presence of noise. However, the flow information fades out quickly across motion boundaries. Dawood and colleagues[43] later advanced the local optical flow algorithm by combining it with a global optical flow algorithm (ie, the method of Horn and Schunck [HS]).[36] The HS algorithm uses the smoothness in flow as the constraint and fills in the missing flow information in inner parts of homogeneous objects from the motion boundaries. The respiratory motion was shown to be reduced in the motion-corrected gated images with the correlation coefficient as the criteria. The combined local and global optical flow algorithm was shown to perform better than the local algorithm.

In the method proposed by Ue and colleagues,[140] the deformation field was defined to consist of control points given as the intersection points of grid lines. By moving each control point, the floating image was deformed. The movement at an arbitrary location in the deformation field was calculated by trilinear interpolation of neighbor control points. In their method, the similarity measure between the reference images and the deformed image was based on the principle that the total activity remains the same after the deformation. An expansion ratio, computed by volumes of tetrahedral, was applied on the deformed image to eliminate the discrepancy between the deformed result and the principle. A smoothness constraint in the deformation served as regularization in the objective function, which was minimized using the simulated annealing algorithm.

Bai and Brady[138,139] proposed B-spline deformable registration algorithms in respiratory motion correction of gated PET images. The control point lattice was assumed as a Markov random field (MRF) to regularize the deformation field. B-splines have the advantage of being smooth functions with explicit derivatives and finite support. Both the gated images and the transformation between them were interpolated using cubic B-spline functions. The MRF was assumed to follow the Gibbs distribution based on the Hammersley-Clifford theorem.[146] Gradient descent was used to minimize the cost function, consisting of the mean squared difference between one image and another deformed image and the regularization term.

Reconstruction Methods

Respiratory motion-compensated image reconstruction methods can be grouped into several categories. One category of methods rebins the PET data by aligning the LORs of each event to the reference position using the estimated motion. Because the event-rebinning method mapping of an LOR is independent of the event location, only rigid or affine motion can be incorporated in the process, which can be a viable approach when focusing on specific tumors or organs.[71] Such an approach was originally developed in brain imaging applications (e.g. Ref.[78]).

A considerably more popular category of methods incorporates the estimated motion within the system matrix for image reconstruction. Nonrigid motion can be applied within the reconstruction process. These techniques use a time/gate-varying system matrix and integrate PET projection data acquired at different time bins into a single comprehensive objective function. The 4D EM formulation (3–4) by Qiao and colleagues,[69] Li and colleagues,[70] and Lamare and colleagues,[71] as discussed in the context of Eq. 3, were originally developed for respiratory motion correction. On advent of simultaneous PET/MR imaging, the recent work by Guerin and colleagues[147] used respiratory motion estimated from tagged MR images to reduce motion blur in whole-body PET studies of torso. This motion correction technique and more recent work by the same group[148] fall into this category as well. The time/gate-varying system matrix method was generalized by Qiao and colleagues[149] to incorporate motions only within a user-defined region of interest. In particular, Li and colleagues[70] considered both a phantom experiment and a clinical study with a pancreatic tumor. They showed increased SNR in images reconstructed with the motion-compensated 4D PET reconstruction over that in images from both regular nongated reconstruction and purely gated reconstruction. The motion artifacts were also clearly reduced in the 4D reconstructed images. **Fig. 4** shows reconstructions obtained using (1) nongated PET, (2) conventional purely gated PET, and (3) the 4D EM algorithm using the entire dataset. The SNR ratios were 2.21, 1.83, and 4.17 for the three approaches.

Reyes and colleagues[150] pursued an approach applicable to nongated datasets. A respiratory motion model constructed from MR images was adapted to each patient's anatomy through affine registrations. The resulting estimated motion was then incorporated into the system matrix of the EM algorithm. Compared with the second category methods, this approach does not require motion estimated beforehand or gating. Nevertheless, the robustness of the model-based motion estimation method given the presence of irregular respiratory patterns as well as interpatient respiratory variations remains questionable. Furthermore, analogous investigations in brain imaging (ie, modeling motion contamination within the system matrix without correction of events)[151] have shown suboptimal convergence properties.

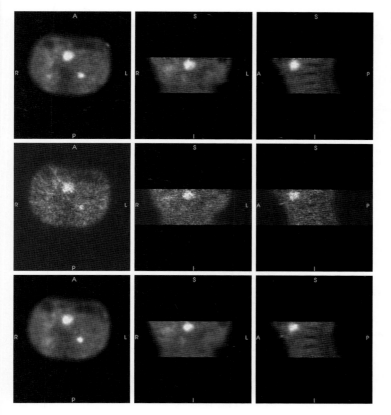

Fig. 4. Reconstructed images of 3D ungated PET obtained by summing all the acquired 4D-PET projections (*top*), conventional 4D PET (*middle*), and model-based 4D PET reconstruction for a clinical study with pancreatic tumor. (*Reprinted from* Li T, Thorndyke B, Schreibmann E, et al. Model-based image reconstruction for four-dimensional PET. Med Phys 2006;33(5):1296; with permission.)

AREAS OF FUTURE RESEARCH

In this section, some areas of research in motion correction are outlined that remain open questions, demanding further inquiries and research:

a. Although theoretic comparisons have been made between postreconstruction and 4D reconstruction methods in which motion is preestimated,[8,9] it remains an open task to theoretically analyze methods in which cardiac or respiratory motion are estimated before or simultaneously with the image reconstruction task. Such analysis might provide insights into further optimization of both categories mentioned earlier, because experimental comparisons have not shown[30,37,42,85,86] a clear advantage of one approach over the other. Development and validation of optimum regularizers, given the distinct spatial resolution properties of motion correction algorithms,[22] is also an area of interest.

b. In dual-gating applications, cardiac versus respiratory gates are commonly treated differently in 4D motion-corrected cardiac imaging applications, wherein the latter are more commonly incorporated within 4D methods, with the former registered and summed after reconstruction.[91,115] However, it is plausible to imagine a combined overall sequence of gates incorporated within the 4D reconstruction framework.[37] Comparison between these two schemes remains an area of interest.

c. Validation and assessment in clinical setting of algorithmic developments in medical imaging is inherently difficult and sometimes unconvincing, particularly when applied to clinical data in the absence of a gold standard, although some approaches to circumvent this limitation have been suggested.[152–154] There is a clear need for guidelines to evaluate image reconstruction and processing techniques in medical imaging research. Task-based assessment of image quality is an emerging field, which will likely help address some of these issues.

d. One of the most active areas of research and development in medical imaging has been the advanced physical anthropomorphic phantoms and computational models that represent the human anatomy[155] and their integration in advanced 4D simulation of time-dependent geometries.[156] Incorporation of accurate models of cardiac and respiratory physiology into the current 4D extended Cardiac-Torso (XCAT) model was a significant step forward to account for inherent cardiac and respiratory motion not considered in the previous

models.[157] Besides providing realistic and flexible simulation of normal cardiac motion, Veress and colleagues[158,159] investigated incorporation of a finite-element mechanical model of the LV to accurately model motion abnormalities such as myocardial ischemia and infarction. Besides simulating cardiac motion in the phantom, this model may be applied as a prior in cardiac motion estimation from emission tomography images to recover the true cardiac motion with twist rather than the apparent motion such as that estimated by optical flow methods.[9]

Likewise, many physical static anthropomorphic phantoms were developed in corporate settings but few dynamic torso phantoms are commercially available and all of them were specifically designed for the assessment of cardiac scanning protocols and ejection fraction calculation software (eg, the dynamic cardiac phantom available from Data Spectrum, Hillsborough, NC). Many academic investigators built dynamic physical phantoms that meet their research needs in cardiac imaging.[160–162] However, similar to commercial systems referred to earlier, virtually none of them incorporate respiratory motion modeling. More advanced technologies allow the construction of dynamic phantoms, allowing modeling of respiratory motion.[163] One interesting design is the platform developed by Fitzpatrick and colleagues,[164] which is capable of programmable irregular longitudinal motion (either artificially generated on a spreadsheet or extracted from respiratory monitoring files) to simulate intrafractional respiratory motion.

SUMMARY

This article summarizes important themes in the emerging field of 4D PET imaging, as applied to cardiac and/or respiratory motion compensation. A wide-ranging choice of techniques are available in research settings but have not yet been used in the clinic. In advanced cardiac and respiratory motion correction schemes, this review has witnessed a general trend to move beyond the noisy images achieved by cardiac-gated and respiratory-gated data which are individually reconstructed, and instead, advanced techniques are seen to make use of novel motion estimation and image reconstruction applications to improve image quality with higher SNR and spatial resolution. There seems to be a general trend toward the use of increasingly sophisticated software for 4D reconstruction in cardiac-gated and respiratory-gated PET imaging. Strategies that endeavor to apply direct 4D PET image reconstruction techniques to motion compensation seem promising but remain to be further refined or constrained to guarantee meaningful reconstructions.

REFERENCES

1. Nehmeh SA, Erdi YE. Respiratory motion in positron emission tomography/computed tomography: a review. Semin Nucl Med 2008;38(3):167–76.
2. Rahmim A, Rousset OG, Zaidi H. Strategies for motion tracking and correction in PET. PET Clin 2007;2:251–66.
3. Klein GJ, Huesman RH. Four-dimensional processing of deformable cardiac PET data. Med Image Anal 2002;6(1):29–46.
4. Dawood M, Buther F, Lang N, et al. Transforming static CT in gated PET/CT studies to multiple respiratory phases. 18th International Conference on Pattern Recognition. Hong Kong, August 20-24, 2006. p. 1026–9.
5. Schafers KP, Dawood M, Lang N, et al. Motion correction in PET/CT. Nuklearmedizin 2005; 44(Suppl 1):S46–50.
6. Thorndyke B, Schreibmann E, Koong A, et al. Reducing respiratory motion artifacts in positron emission tomography through retrospective stacking. Med Phys 2006;33(7):2632–41.
7. Le Meunier L, Slomka PJ, Dey D, et al. Motion frozen F-18-FDG cardiac PET. J Nucl Cardiol 2011;18(2):259–66.
8. Asma E, Manjeshwar R, Thielemans K. Theoretical comparison of motion correction techniques for PET image reconstruction. IEEE Nuclear Science Symposium Conference Record; San Diego, CA, 29 October - 4 November, 2006. p. 1762–7.
9. Chun SY, Fessler JY. Noise properties of motion-compensated tomographic image reconstruction methods. IEEE Trans Med Imaging in press.
10. Rahmim A, Tang J, Zaidi H. Four-dimensional (4D) image reconstruction strategies in dynamic PET: beyond conventional independent frame reconstruction. Med Phys 2009;36(8):3654–70.
11. Grotus N, Reader AJ, Stute S, et al. Fully 4D list-mode reconstruction applied to respiratory-gated PET scans. Phys Med Biol 2009;54(6): 1705–21.
12. Verhaeghe J, D'Asseler Y, Staelens S, et al. Reconstruction for gated dynamic cardiac PET imaging using a tensor product spline basis. IEEE Trans Nucl Sci 2007;54(1):80–91.
13. Niu XF, Yang YY, Wernick MN. 4D reconstruction of cardiac images using temporal Fourier basis functions. Presented at 15th IEEE International Conference on Image Processing. vols. 1–5. San Diego, CA, October 12-15, 2008. p. 2944–7.
14. O'Dell WG, Moore CC, Hunter WC, et al. Three-dimensional myocardial deformations: calculation with displacement field fitting to tagged MR images. Radiology 1995;195(3):829–35.
15. Di Carli MF, Dorbala S, Meserve J, et al. Clinical myocardial perfusion PET/CT. J Nucl Med 2007; 48(5):783–93.
16. Hutchins GD, Caraher JM, Raylman RR. A region of interest strategy for minimizing resolution distortions in quantitative myocardial PET studies. J Nucl Med 1992;33(6):1243–50.
17. Nichols K, Lefkowitz D, Faber T, et al. Echocardiographic validation of gated SPECT ventricular function measurements. J Nucl Med 2000;41(8): 1308–14.
18. Visvikis D, Lamare F, Bruyant P, et al. Correction de mouvement respiratoire en TEP/TDM. Med Nucl 2007;31(4):153–9 [in French].
19. Pombo JF, Troy BL, Russell RO Jr. Left ventricular volumes and ejection fraction by echocardiography. Circulation 1971;43(4):480–90.
20. Dumesnil JG, Shoucri RM, Laurenceau JL, et al. A mathematical model of the dynamic geometry of the intact left ventricle and its application to clinical data. Circulation 1979;59(5):1024–34.
21. Holman ER, Buller VG, de Roos A, et al. Detection and quantification of dysfunctional myocardium by magnetic resonance imaging. A new three-dimensional method for quantitative wall-thickening analysis. Circulation 1997;95(4):924–31.
22. Cao Z, Gilland D, Mair B, et al. Simultaneous reconstruction and 3D motion estimation for gated myocardial emission CT using the 4D NCAT phantom [abstract]. J Nucl Med 2003; 44(5):9P.
23. Gilland DR, Mair BA, Bowsher JE, et al. Simultaneous reconstruction and motion estimation for gated cardiac ECT. IEEE Trans Nucl Sci 2002; 49(5):2344–9.
24. Gravier E, Yang Y, King MA, et al. Fully 4D motion-compensated reconstruction of cardiac SPECT images. Phys Med Biol 2006;51(18):4603–19.
25. Mair BA, Gilland DR, Sun J. Estimation of images and nonrigid deformations in gated emission CT. IEEE Trans Med Imaging 2006;25(9): 1130–44.
26. Zerhouni EA, Parish DM, Rogers WJ, Yang A, Shapiro EP. Human heart: tagging with MR imaging-a method for noninvasive assessment of myocardial motion. Radiology 1988;169(1): 59–63.
27. Axel L, Dougherty L. MR imaging of motion with spatial modulation of magnetization. Radiology 1989;171(3):841–5.
28. Axel L, Montillo A, Kim D. Tagged magnetic resonance imaging of the heart: a survey. Med Image Anal 2005;9(4):376–93.

29. Young AA, Kraitchman DL, Dougherty L, et al. Tracking and finite-element analysis of stripe deformation in magnetic-resonance tagging. IEEE Trans Med Imaging 1995;14(3):413–21.

30. Park J, Metaxas D, Young AA, et al. Deformable models with parameter functions for cardiac motion analysis from tagged MRI data. IEEE Trans Med Imaging 1996;15(3):278–89.

31. Ozturk C, McVeigh ER. Four-dimensional B-spline based motion analysis of tagged MR images: introduction and in vivo validation. Phys Med Biol 2000; 45(6):1683–702.

32. Osman NF, McVeigh ER, Prince JL. Imaging heart motion using harmonic phase MRI. IEEE Trans Med Imaging 2000;19(3):186–202.

33. Delso G, Furst S, Jakoby B, et al. Performance measurements of the Siemens mMR integrated whole-body PET/MR scanner. J Nucl Med 2011; 52(12):1914–22.

34. Wehrl HF, Sauter AW, Judenhofer MS, et al. Combined PET/MR imaging–technology and applications. Technol Cancer Res Treat 2010;9(1): 5–20.

35. Petibon Y, Ouyang J, Zhu X, et al. MR-based motion compensation in simultaneous cardiac PET-MR. J Nucl Med 2012;53(Suppl 1):108.

36. Horn BK, Schunck BG. Determining optical flow. Artif Intell 1981;17(1–3):185–203.

37. Mailloux GE, Bleau A, Bertrand M, et al. Computer-analysis of heart motion from two-dimensional echocardiograms. IEEE Trans Biomed Eng 1987; 34(5):356–64.

38. Amartur SC, Vesselle HJ. A new approach to study cardiac motion: the optical flow of cine MR images. Magn Reson Med 1993;29(1):59–67.

39. Song SM, Leahy RM. Computation of 3-D velocity fields from 3-D cine CT images of a human heart. IEEE Trans Med Imaging 1991;10(3):295–306.

40. Zhou ZY, Synolakis CE, Leahy RM, et al. Calculation of 3D internal displacement-fields from 3D X-ray computer tomographic-images. Proc R Soc London A 1995;449(1937):537–54.

41. Love AE. A treatise on the mathematical theory of elasticity. Cambridge (United Kingdom): Cambridge University Press; 1927.

42. Cao Z, Gilland DR, Mair BA, et al. Three-dimensional motion estimation with image reconstruction for gated cardiac ECT. IEEE Trans Nucl Sci 2003; 50(3):384–8.

43. Dawood M, Buther F, Jiang X, et al. Respiratory motion correction in 3-D PET data with advanced optical flow algorithms. IEEE Trans Med Imaging 2008;27(8):1164–75.

44. Beauchemin SS, Barron JL. The computation of optical flow. ACM Comput Surv 1995;27(3):433–66.

45. Barron JL, Fleet DJ, Beauchemin SS, et al. Performance of optical flow techniques. Proceedings Computer Vision and Pattern Recognition. Champaign, IL, June 15–18, 1992. p. 236–42.

46. Tang J, Segars WP, Lee TS, et al. Quantitative study of cardiac motion estimation and abnormality classification in emission computed tomography. Med Eng Phys 2011;33(5):563–72.

47. Slomka PJ, Nishina H, Berman DS, et al. "Motion-frozen" display and quantification of myocardial perfusion. J Nucl Med 2004;45(7):1128–34.

48. Brankov JG, Yang Y, Narayanan MV, et al. Motion-compensated 4D processing of gated SPECT perfusion studies. IEEE Nuclear Science Symposium Conference Record, 2002. Norfolk (VA), November 10–16, 2002. p. 1380–4.

49. Brankov JG, Yang Y, Wernick MN. Tomographic image reconstruction based on a content-adaptive mesh model. IEEE Trans Med Imaging 2004;23(2):202–12.

50. Marin T, Brankov JG. Deformable left-ventricle mesh model for motion-compensated filtering in cardiac gated SPECT. Med Phys 2010;37(10):5471–81.

51. Brankov JG, Yang Y, Wernick MN. Spatiotemporal processing of gated cardiac SPECT images using deformable mesh modeling. Med Phys 2005; 32(9):2839–49.

52. Jacobson M, Levkovitz R, Ben-Tal A, et al. Enhanced 3D PET OSEM reconstruction using inter-update Metz filtering. Phys Med Biol 2000;45(8):2417–39.

53. Mustafovic S, Thielemans K. Object dependency of resolution in reconstruction algorithms with inter-iteration filtering applied to PET data. IEEE Trans Med Imaging 2004;23(4):433–46.

54. Kadrmas DJ, Gullberg GT. 4D maximum a posteriori reconstruction in dynamic SPECT using a compartmental model-based prior. Phys Med Biol 2001;46(5):1553–74.

55. Reader AJ, Matthews JC, Sureau FC, et al. Iterative kinetic parameter estimation within fully 4D PET image reconstruction. IEEE Nuclear Science Symposium Conference Record. San Diego, CA, 29 October - 4 November, 2006. p. 1752–6.

56. Geman S, McClure DE. Statistical methods for tomographic image reconstruction. Bull Int Stat Inst 1987;52(4):5–21.

57. Chinn G, Huang SC. A general class of preconditioners for statistical iterative reconstruction of emission computed tomography. IEEE Trans Med Imaging 1997;16(1):1–10.

58. Shepp LA, Vardi Y. Maximum likelihood reconstruction for emission tomography. IEEE Trans Med Imaging 1982;1:113–22.

59. Lange K, Carson R. EM reconstruction algorithms for emission and transmission tomography. J Comput Assist Tomogr 1984;8(2):306–16.

60. Green PJ. Bayesian reconstructions from emission tomography data using a modified EM algorithm. IEEE Trans Med Imaging 1990;9:84–93.

61. Gravier EJ, Yang Y. Motion-compensated reconstruction of tomographic image sequences. IEEE Trans Nucl Sci 2005;52(1):51–6.

62. Gravier E, Yang YY, Jin MW. Tomographic reconstruction of dynamic cardiac image sequences. IEEE Trans Image Process 2007;16(4):932–42.

63. Lalush DS, Lin C, Tsui BM. A priori motion models for four-dimensional reconstruction in gated cardiac SPECT. IEEE Nuclear Science Symposium Conference Record, 1996. Anaheim (CA), November 2–9, 1996. p. 1923–7.

64. Lalush DS, Tsui BM. Block-iterative techniques for fast 4D reconstruction using a priori motion models in gated cardiac SPECT. Phys Med Biol 1998;43(4): 875–86.

65. Lee TS, Lautamaki R, Higuchi T, et al. Task-based human observer study for evaluation and optimization of 3D & 4D image reconstruction methods for gated myocardial perfusion SPECT. J Nucl Med 2009;50(Suppl 2):524.

66. Lee TS, Bengel F, Tsui BM. Task-based human observer study for evaluation of 4D MAP-RBI-EM method for gated myocardial perfusion SPECT. J Nucl Med 2008;49(Suppl 1):153P.

67. Lee TS, Segars WP, Tsui BM. Study of parameters characterizing space-time Gibbs priors for 4D MAP-RBI-EM in gated myocardial perfusion SPECT. IEEE Nuclear Science Symposium Conference Record. Wyndham El Conquistador, Puerto Rico, October 23–29, 2005. p. 2124–8.

68. Tang J, Lee TS, He X, et al. Comparison of 3D OS-EM and 4D MAP-RBI-EM reconstruction algorithms for cardiac motion abnormality classification using a motion observer. IEEE Trans Nucl Sci 2010; 57(5):2571–7.

69. Qiao F, Pan T, Clark JW Jr, et al. A motion-incorporated reconstruction method for gated PET studies. Phys Med Biol 2006;51(15):3769–83.

70. Li T, Thorndyke B, Schreibmann E, et al. Model-based image reconstruction for four-dimensional PET. Med Phys 2006;33(5):1288–98.

71. Lamare F, Cresson T, Savean J, et al. Respiratory motion correction for PET oncology applications using affine transformation of list mode data. Phys Med Biol 2007;52(1):121–40.

72. Tang J, Bengel F, Rahmim A. Cardiac motion-corrected quantitative dynamic Rb-82 PET imaging. J Nucl Med 2010;51(Suppl 2):123.

73. Hebert TJ, Leahy R. Fast methods for including attenuation in the EM algorithm. IEEE Trans Nucl Sci 1990;37(2):754–8.

74. Mumcuoglu EU, Leahy R, Cherry SR, et al. Fast gradient-based methods for Bayesian reconstruction of transmission and emission PET images. IEEE Trans Med Imaging 1994;13(4):687–701.

75. Reader AJ, Ally S, Bakatselos F, et al. One-pass list-mode EM algorithm for high-resolution 3-D PET image reconstruction into large arrays. IEEE Trans Nucl Sci 2002;49(3):693–9.

76. Daube-Witherspoon M, Yan Y, Green M, et al. Correction for motion distortion in PET by dynamic monitoring of patient position [abstract]. J Nucl Med 1990;31:816.

77. Menke M, Atkins MS, Buckley KR. Compensation methods for head motion detected during PET imaging. IEEE Trans Nucl Sci 1996;43(1):310–7.

78. Bloomfield PM, Spinks TJ, Reed J, et al. The design and implementation of a motion correction scheme for neurological PET. Phys Med Biol 2003;48(8):959–78.

79. Rahmim A, Dinelle K, Cheng JC, et al. Accurate event-driven motion compensation in high-resolution PET incorporating scattered and random events. IEEE Trans Med Imaging 2008; 27(8):1018–33.

80. Rahmim A, Bloomfield P, Houle S, et al. Motion compensation in histogram-mode and list-mode EM reconstructions: beyond the event-driven approach. IEEE Trans Nucl Sci 2004;51:2588–96.

81. Qi J, Huesman RH. List mode reconstruction for PET with motion compensation: a simulation study. Proceedings IEEE International Symposium on Biomedical Imaging, 2002. Washington, DC. July 7–10, 2002. p. 413–6.

82. Carson RE, Barker WC, Liow JS, et al. Design of a motion-compensation OSEM list-mode algorithm for resolution-recovery reconstruction for the HRRT. IEEE Nuclear Science Symposium Conference Record, 2003. Portland (OR). October 19–25, 2003. p. 3281–5.

83. Qi J. Calculation of the sensitivity image in list-mode reconstruction for PET. IEEE Trans Nucl Sci 2006;53(5):2746–51.

84. Gilland DR, Mair BA, Sun J. Joint 4D reconstruction and motion estimation in gated cardiac ECT. Proceedings of the International Meeting on Fully Three-Dimensional Image Reconstruction in Radiology and Nuclear Medicine. Salt Lake City (UT), July 6–9, 2005. p. 303–6.

85. Jacobson MW, Fessler JA. Joint estimation of image and deformation parameters in motion-corrected PET. IEEE Nuclear Science Symposium Conference Record. 2003. p. 3290–4.

86. Jacobson MW, Fessler JA. Joint estimation of respiratory motion and activity in 4D PET using CT side information. Presented at 3rd IEEE International Symposium on Biomedical Imaging: Nano to Macro. Arlington, VA, April 6–9, 2006. p. 275–8.

87. Blume M, Martinez-Moller A, Keil A, et al. Joint reconstruction of image and motion in gated positron emission tomography. IEEE Trans Med Imaging 2010;29(11):1892–906.

88. Livieratos L, Rajappan K, Stegger L, et al. Respiratory gating of cardiac PET data in list-mode

acquisition. Eur J Nucl Med Mol Imaging 2006; 33(5):584–8.

89. Rahmim A, Tang J, Ay MR, et al. 4D respiratory motion-corrected Rb-82 myocardial perfusion PET imaging. IEEE Nuclear Science Symposium Conference Record. Knoxville, TN, 30 October - 6 November, 2010. p. 3312–6.

90. Park MJ, Chen S, Lee TS, et al. Generation and evaluation of a simultaneous cardiac and respiratory gated Rb-82 PET simulation. Presented at IEEE Nuclear Science Symposium and Medical Imaging Conference (NSS/MIC). Valencia, Spain, October 23–29, 2011. p. 3327–30.

91. Chen S, Bravo P, Lodge M, et al. Four-dimensional PET image reconstruction with respiratory and cardiac motion compensation from list-mode data. J Nucl Med 2012;53(1_MeetingAbstracts):106.

92. Teras M, Kokki T, Durand-Schaefer N, et al. Dual-gated cardiac PET–clinical feasibility study. Eur J Nucl Med Mol Imaging 2010;37(3):505–16.

93. Kreissl MC, Stout D, Silverman RW, et al. Heart and respiratory gating of cardiac microPET (R)/CT studies in mice. IEEE Nuclear Science Symposium Conference Record. vols. 1–7. Rome, Italy, October 19–22, 2004. p. 3877–9.

94. Klein GJ, Reutter BW, Ho MH, et al. Real-time system for respiratory-cardiac gating in positron tomography. IEEE Trans Nucl Sci 1998;45(4): 2139–43.

95. Lang N, Dawood M, Büther F, et al. Organ movement reduction in PET/CT using dual-gated list-mode acquisition. Z Med Phys 2006;16(1):93–100.

96. Martinez-Möller A, Zikic D, Botnar RM, et al. Dual cardiac/respiratory gated PET: implementation and results from a feasibility study. Eur J Nuc Med Mol Imaging 2007;34(9):1447–54.

97. Yang Y, Rendig S, Siegel S, et al. Cardiac PET imaging in mice with simultaneous cardiac and respiratory gating. Phys Med Biol 2005;50(13): 2979–89.

98. Schafers KP, Lang N, Stegger L, et al. Gated list-mode acquisition with the QuadHIDAC animal PET to image mouse hearts. Z Med Phys 2006; 16(1):60–6.

99. Klein GJ, Reutter RW, Huesman RH. Four-dimensional affine registration models for respiratory-gated PET. IEEE Trans Nucl Sci 2001;48(3):756–60.

100. Le Meunier L, Slomka P, Fermin J, et al. Motion frozen of dual gated (cardiac and respiratory) PET images. J Nucl Med 2009;50(2_MeetingAbstracts): 1474.

101. Livieratos L, Stegger L, Bloomfield PM, et al. Rigid-body transformation of list-mode projection data for respiratory motion correction in cardiac PET. Phys Med Biol 2005;14:3313–22.

102. Bruyant PP, King MA, Pretorius PH. Correction of the respiratory motion of the heart by tracking of the center of mass of thresholded projections: a simulation study using the dynamic MCAT phantom. IEEE Trans Nucl Sci 2002;49(5):2159–66.

103. Segars WP, Mori S, Chen GT, et al. Modeling respiratory motion variations in the 4D NCAT phantom. IEEE Nuclear Science Symposium Conference Record. Honolulu, Hawaii, 28 October - 3 November, 2007. NSS '07. IEEE. 2007. p. 2677–9.

104. Korin HW, Ehman RL, Riederer SJ, et al. Respiratory kinematics of the upper abdominal organs–a quantitative study. Magn Reson Med 1992; 23(1):172–8.

105. Hoffman EA, Ritman EL. Heart-lung interaction: effect on regional lung air content and total heart volume. Ann Biomed Eng 1987;15(3–4):241–57.

106. Andersen K, Vik-Mo H. Effects of spontaneous respiration on left ventricular function assessed by echocardiography. Circulation 1984;69(5): 874–9.

107. Qi J, Leahy RM, Chinghan H, et al. Fully 3D Bayesian image reconstruction for the ECAT EXACT HR+. IEEE Trans Nucl Sci 1998;45(3): 1096–103.

108. Panin VY, Kehren F, Michel C, et al. Fully 3-D PET reconstruction with system matrix derived from point source measurements. IEEE Trans Med Imaging 2006;25(7):907–21.

109. Panin VY, Kehren F, Rothfuss H, et al. PET reconstruction with system matrix derived from point source measurements. IEEE Trans Nucl Sci 2006; 53(1):152–9.

110. Alessio AM, Kinahan PE, Lewellen TK. Modeling and incorporation of system response functions in 3-D whole body PET. IEEE Trans Med Imaging 2006;25(7):828–37.

111. Rahmim A, Tang J, Lodge MA, et al. Analytic system matrix resolution modeling in PET: an application to Rb-82 cardiac imaging. Phys Med Biol 2008;53(21):5947–65.

112. Alessio AM, Stearns CW, Shan T, et al. Application and evaluation of a measured spatially variant system model for PET image reconstruction. IEEE Trans Med Imaging 2010;29(3):938–49.

113. Le Meunier L, Slomka PJ, Dey D, et al. Enhanced definition PET for cardiac imaging. J Nucl Cardiol 2010;17(3):414–26.

114. Buhler P, Just U, Will E, et al. An accurate method for correction of head movement in PET. IEEE Trans Med Imaging 2004;23(9):1176–85.

115. Tang J, Hall N, Rahmim A. MRI assisted motion correction in dual-gated 5D myocardial perfusion PET imaging. IEEE Nuclear Science Symposium Conference Record 2012, in press.

116. Bengel FM, Higuchi T, Javadi MS, et al. Cardiac positron emission tomography. J Am Coll Cardiol 2009;54(1):1–15.

117. Lodge M, Bengel F. Methodology for quantifying absolute myocardial perfusion with PET and SPECT. Curr Cardiol Rep 2007;9(2):121–8.

118. Uren NG, Melin JA, De Bruyne B, et al. Relation between myocardial blood flow and the severity of coronary-artery stenosis. N Engl J Med 1994; 330(25):1782–8.

119. Parkash R, DeKemp RA, Ruddy TD, et al. Potential utility of rubidium 82 PET quantification in patients with 3-vessel coronary artery disease. J Nucl Cardiol 2004;11(4):440–9.

120. Guethlin M, Kasel AM, Coppenrath K, et al. Delayed response of myocardial flow reserve to lipid-lowering therapy with fluvastatin. Circulation 1999;99(4):475–81.

121. Huggins GS, Pasternak RC, Alpert NM, et al. Effects of short-term treatment of hyperlipidemia on coronary vasodilator function and myocardial perfusion in regions having substantial impairment of baseline dilator reverse. Circulation 1998;98(13):1291–6.

122. Schindler TH, Nitzsche EU, Schelbert HR, et al. Positron emission tomography-measured abnormal responses of myocardial blood flow to sympathetic stimulation are associated with the risk of developing cardiovascular events. J Am Coll Cardiol 2005;45(9):1505–12.

123. Schindler TH, Nitzsche E, Magosaki N, et al. Regional myocardial perfusion defects during exercise, as assessed by three dimensional integration of morphology and function, in relation to abnormal endothelium dependent vasoreactivity of the coronary microcirculation. Heart 2003;89(5):517–26.

124. Schachinger V, Britten MB, Zeiher AM. Prognostic impact of coronary vasodilator dysfunction on adverse long-term outcome of coronary heart disease. Circulation 2000;101(16):1899–906.

125. Tsoumpas C, Turkheimer FE, Thielemans K. A survey of approaches for direct parametric image reconstruction in emission tomography. Med Phys 2008;35(9):3963–71.

126. Farncombe TH, Feng B, King MA, et al. Investigating acquisition protocols for gated, dynamic myocardial imaging in PET and SPECT. 2003 IEEE Nuclear Science Symposium Conference Record. vols. 1–5. Rome, Italy, October 19–22, 2004. p. 3272–5.

127. Feng B, Pretorius PH, Farncombe TH, et al. Simultaneous assessment of cardiac perfusion and function using 5-dimensional imaging with Tc-99m teboroxime. J Nucl Cardiol 2006;13(3):354–61.

128. Jin MW, Yang YY, King MA. Reconstruction of dynamic gated cardiac SPECT. Med Phys 2006; 33(11):4384–94.

129. Niu XF, Yang YY, Jin MW, et al. Regularized fully 5D reconstruction of cardiac gated dynamic SPECT images. IEEE Trans Nucl Sci 2010;57(3): 1085–95.

130. Niu XF, Yang YY, Wernick MN. Direct reconstruction of parametric images from cardiac gated dynamic SPECT data. Presented at 18th IEEE International Conference on Image Processing (ICIP). Brussels, Belgium, September 11–14, 2011. p. 453–6.

131. Shi YG, Karl WC. A multiphase level set method for tomographic reconstruction of dynamic objects. Proceedings of the 2003 IEEE Workshop on Statistical Signal Processing. St. Louis, Missouri, September 28 - October 1, 2003. p. 182–5.

132. Shi YG, Karl WC. Level set methods for dynamic tomography. Presented at 2nd IEEE International Symposium on Biomedical Imaging: Macro to Nano. vols. 1 and 2. Arlington, VA, April 15–18, 2004. p. 620–3.

133. Fitzpatrick GM, Wells RG. Simulation study of respiratory-induced errors in cardiac positron emission tomography/computed tomography. Med Phys 2006;33(8):2888–95.

134. Le Meunier L, Maass-Moreno R, Carrasquillo JA, et al. PET/CT imaging: effect of respiratory motion on apparent myocardial uptake. J Nucl Cardiol 2006;13(6):821–30.

135. Pan T, Mawlawi O, Nehmeh SA, et al. Attenuation correction of PET images with respiration-averaged CT images in PET/CT. J Nucl Med 2005; 46(9):1481–7.

136. Nagel CC, Bosmans G, Dekker AL, et al. Phased attenuation correction in respiration correlated computed tomography/positron emitted tomography. Med Phys 2006;33(6):1840–7.

137. Lamare F, Ledesma Carbayo MJ, Cresson T, et al. List-mode-based reconstruction for respiratory motion correction in PET using non-rigid body transformations. Phys Med Biol 2007;52(17):5187–204.

138. Bai W, Brady M. Regularized B-spline deformable registration for respiratory motion correction in PET images. Phys Med Biol 2009;54(9):2719–36.

139. Bai W, Brady M. Motion correction and attenuation correction for respiratory gated PET images. IEEE Trans Med Imaging 2011;30(2):351–65.

140. Ue H, Haneishi H, Iwanaga H, et al. Nonlinear motion correction of respiratory-gated lung SPECT images. IEEE Trans Med Imaging 2006; 25(4):486–95.

141. Fin L, Bailly P, Daouk J, et al. Motion correction based on an appropriate system matrix for statistical reconstruction of respiratory-correlated PET acquisitions. Comput Methods Programs Biomed 2009;96(3):e1–9.

142. Dawood M, Lang N, Jiang X, et al. Lung motion correction on respiratory gated 3-D PET/CT images. IEEE Trans Med Imaging 2006;25(4):476–85.

143. Liu C, Alessio AM, Kinahan PE. Respiratory motion correction for quantitative PET/CT using all detected events with internal-external motion correlation. Med Phys 2011;38(5):2715–23.

144. Chan C, Jing X, Fung EK, et al. Event-by-event respiratory motion correction for PET with 3-dimensional internal-external motion correlation, IEEE Nuclear Science Symposium Conference Record, (Anaheim, CA, 29 Oct – 3 Nov 2012), in press.

145. Lucas BD, Kanade T. An iterative image registration technique with an application to stereo vision. Presented at DARPA Image Understanding Workshop. Vancouver, British Columbia, Canada, August 24–28, 1981. p. 121–30.

146. Clifford P. Markov random fields in statistics. In: Grimmett G, Welsh DJ, editors. Disorder in physical systems. Clarendon (TX): Oxford; 1990. p. 19–32.

147. Guerin B, Cho S, Chun SY, et al. Nonrigid PET motion compensation in the lower abdomen using simultaneous tagged-MRI and PET imaging. Med Phys 2011;38(6):3025–38.

148. Chun SY, Reese TG, Ouyang J, et al. MRI-based nonrigid motion correction in simultaneous PET/MRI. J Nucl Med, in press.

149. Qiao F, Pan T, Clark JW, et al. Region of interest motion compensation for PET image reconstruction. Phys Med Biol 2007;52(10):2675–89.

150. Reyes M, Malandain G, Koulibaly PM, et al. Model-based respiratory motion compensation for emission tomography image reconstruction. Phys Med Biol 2007;52(12):3579–600.

151. Rahmim A, Cheng JC, Dinelle K, et al. System matrix modelling of externally tracked motion. Nucl Med Commun 2008;29(6):574–81.

152. Kupinski MA, Hoppin JW, Clarkson E, et al. Estimation in medical imaging without a gold standard. Acad Radiol 2002;9(3):290–7.

153. Hoppin JW, Kupinski MA, Wilson DW, et al. Evaluating estimation techniques in medical imaging without a gold standard: experimental validation. Proceedings of SPIE 2003;5034:230–7.

154. Lehmann T. From plastic to gold: a unified classification scheme for reference standards in medical image processing. Presented at Medical Imaging 2002: Image Processing. San Diego (CA), February 24–28, 2002. p. 1819–27.

155. Zaidi H, Xu XG. Computational anthropomorphic models of the human anatomy: the path to realistic Monte Carlo modeling in medical imaging. Annu Rev Biomed Eng 2007;9(1):471–500.

156. Paganetti H. Four-dimensional Monte Carlo simulation of time-dependent geometries. Phys Med Biol 2004;49(6):N75–81.

157. Segars WP, Tsui BM. MCAT to XCAT: the evolution of 4D computerized phantoms for imaging research. Proc IEEE 2009;97(12):1954–68.

158. Veress AI, Segars WP, Tsui BM, et al. Incorporation of a left ventricle finite element model defining infarction into the XCAT imaging phantom. IEEE Trans Med Imaging 2011;30(4):915–27.

159. Veress AI, Segars WP, Weiss JA, et al. Normal and pathological NCAT image and phantom data based on physiologically realistic left ventricle finite-element models. IEEE Trans Med Imaging 2006;25(12):1604–16.

160. De Bondt P, Claessens T, Rys B, et al. Accuracy of 4 different algorithms for the analysis of tomographic radionuclide ventriculography using a physical, dynamic 4-chamber cardiac phantom. J Nucl Med 2005;46(1):165–71.

161. Begemann PG, van Stevendaal U, Manzke R, et al. Evaluation of spatial and temporal resolution for ECG-gated 16-row multidetector CT using a dynamic cardiac phantom. Eur Radiol 2005;15(5):1015–26.

162. Al Hamwi A. Construction and optimal design of a dynamic heart phantom for simulation of motion artefacts in PET scan. Biomed Tech (Berl) 2002;47(Suppl 1 Pt 2):810–1 [in German].

163. Kashani R, Hub M, Kessler ML, et al. Technical note: a physical phantom for assessment of accuracy of deformable alignment algorithms. Med Phys 2007;34(7):2785–8.

164. Fitzpatrick MJ, Starkschall G, Balter P, et al. A novel platform simulating irregular motion to enhance assessment of respiration-correlated radiation therapy procedures. J Appl Clin Med Phys 2005;6(1):13–21.

Clinical Impact of Cardiac-Gated PET Imaging

Stephan G. Nekolla, PhD*, Julia Dinges, MD,
Christoph Rischpler, MD

KEYWORDS

• Positron emission tomography • Hybrid imaging • Cardiac gating • Viability • Perfusion

KEY POINTS

- Gated positron emission tomography has been validated in numerous studies over the last decade and shows clear incremental value in both ischemia and viability imaging.
- Modern positron emission tomography/computed tomography systems with list mode acquisitions offer powerful and convenient means for dynamic and gated positron emission tomography imaging in the clinical arena of multimodality imaging.
- The integration of quantitative, regional, multiparameter information will further enhance the diagnostic quality of positron emission tomography cardiac imaging.

INTRODUCTION

The capability of positron emission tomography (PET) to generate images that are triggered to the electrocardiogram (ECG) is a powerful extension to its already documented expertise in cardiac imaging. This review discusses the historical development, technical aspects, and those applications in which incremental value is achieved.

In the last decade, clinical PET use increased markedly. Because of the increasing application in oncologic imaging, the number of hybrid PET/computed tomography (CT) devices showed an impressive growth. The increased availability of those scanners resulted in the opportunity to use these scanners also for cardiac imaging.[1,2] This development is expected to continue as new ^{18}F labeled PET perfusion agents enter the field[3–5] that supersede the need for a local cyclotron or cost-intensive generators requiring a certain patient throughput.

In general, PET myocardial perfusion imaging (MPI) is generally considered the gold standard for noninvasive estimation of absolute myocardial blood flow.[6] The second major application is the assessment of myocardial viability by PET with ^{18}F fluordeoxyglucose (^{18}F FDG-PET), which is also considered the gold standard.[7,8] Several studies over 2 decades showed the value of ^{18}F FDG-PET imaging to identify those patients who most likely would benefit from revascularization.[7,9,10] Furthermore, using more specific tracers, it is expected that the role of PET role will increase in the future for early detection and prevention of disease.[11]

In almost all the aforementioned studies, PET data were acquired either in a static mode after the radiopharmaceutical reached an equilibrium phase and the relative tracer distribution was analyzed either visually or quantitatively. The other approach used was dynamic imaging to extract physiologic variable such as absolute myocardial blood flow or other metabolic parameters. However, the generation of cardiac images acquired together with the ECG to assess regional and global myocardial function is also possible.

Disclosure: All authors declare that there are no conflicts of interest to disclose within the context of this manuscript.

Nuklearmedizinische Klinik der Technischen Universität München, Ismaningerstr. 22, D 81675 München, Germany

* Corresponding author.

E-mail address: stephan.nekolla@tum.de

PET Clin 8 (2013) 69–79

http://dx.doi.org/10.1016/j.cpet.2012.10.002

THE ROAD TO GATED PET

The fundamental idea dates back to the 1970s[12] and is one of the earliest examples of functional imaging using nuclear scintigraphy with substantial clinical impact.[13–15] Basically, equilibrium-gated blood pool imaging allows the visualization of the contracting myocardial chambers after the vascular pool is marked with a radiopharmaceutical such as human serum albumin labeled with technetium Tc 99m or red blood cells tagged with the same isotope. Planar images are acquired with high frame rates together with the ECG and, after completion of the examination, are sorted and summed into typically 16 gates, allowing for a sophisticated analysis. This approach with blood pool agents was later extended to single photon emission computed tomography (SPECT) imaging,[16] which allowed for an improved assessment of myocardial function, because the effects from overlapping structures could be avoided.[17–19] Whereas equilibrium-gated blood pool agents focused on the contrast of lumen versus myocardium, perfusion agents such as Tl-201 assessed the myocardium directly. Combining this with injection during a stress test, the assessment of ischemia and thus coronary artery disease became one of the most successful imaging approaches.[20] Consequently, the delineation of myocardial contractility was investigated as well. However, using SPECT imaging,[21] the moderate image quality of Tl-201 made the acquisition of gated studies complicated.

This situation changed with the advent of technetium Tc 99m–labeled myocardial perfusion tracers.[22] The higher energy of the emitted photon (140 keV vs 70 keV) and the shorter half-life (6 h vs 73 h) resulted in significantly better image quality and also lower radiation exposure of the patient. Consequently, ECG-triggered cardiac MPI scans became feasible and are today used routinely to assess regional and global function as a clinically highly relevant side product to myocardial perfusion.

CARDIAC-GATED PET IMAGING: TECHNICAL CONSIDERATIONS

Compared with SPECT imaging, PET allows the quantitative determination of regional tracer distributions. Calibration procedures using homogeneous phantoms filled with positron-emitting substances correct for different sensitivities of the detectors and the attached photomultipliers. In addition, the distribution of photon attenuating tissue is used to correct the measured emission signal. In conventional PET, these attenuation data were acquired with lengthy transmission scans using rotating, external source cameras. Today, attenuation correction in PET/CT systems is based on comparatively much shorter CT transmission scans. However, proper attenuation correction is a prerequisite to PET and especially PET/CT—including gated PET/CT. Inconsistencies between emission and transmission data can lead to significant artifacts, and strict quality control is mandatory.[23–26] This is in clear difference to cardiac SPECT, in which attenuation correction appears to be less of a problem. To improve disease detection, this was an extensive area of research in the last 2 decades, but with the recent advance of fast SPECT devices, the interest appears to be reduced.[27]

Similar to dynamic imaging, cardiac gating was used as early as 1979 by Hoffman and colleagues[28] using several radiopharmaceuticals and used to be a standard feature in PET-only tomographs.[29–32] However, like dynamic imaging, this option initially was not always available in PET/CT systems because the focus was on oncologic imaging. However, the success of cardiac gating in SPECT imaging led the industry to necessary implementations for this technique, which provides valuable information at practically no extra cost during the acquisition. In addition, the latest generation of PET/CT systems replaced conventional detector materials (eg, bismuth germanium oxide [BGO]) with materials such as lutetium oxyorthosilicate capable of increased light output for gated imaging due to their increased sensitivity and decreased light decay.[33–35] This clearly improved the acquisition of gated studies.

The implementation of cardiac-gated PET is similar to that of SPECT: Parallel to the registration of all coincidence events, the physiologic ECG signal is registered. Thus, the association of a given coincidence event with myocardial contraction is possible. Typically, the ECG signal is measured with electrodes attached to the patient and fed into external devices or integrated hardware in the scanner gantry. For prospective ECG gating (which was the standard in conventional PET devices), the number of cardiac phases after (forward gating) or before (backward gating) the detected R wave must be defined. Then, in the emission scan, the corresponding annihilation events are sorted into the predefined sinogram buffers. After the end of the data acquisition, the sinograms are normalized and ideally corrected for misalignment, scatter, and attenuation and image reconstruction is performed. Depending on the level of sophistication of the vendor's implementation, parameters such as the minimal or maximal R-wave to R-wave interval can be specified before the acquisition. In case of cardiac arrhythmias, those beats outside of the R-wave to R-wave interval are rejected or collected in a bad beat buffer. With the availability of list mode acquisitions in which all events are stored, more flexibility and sophisticated algorithms can be used retrospectively as discussed in one of the following sections.

GATED PET: VALIDATION AND APPLICATIONS

Validation studies over almost a decade have found a good agreement of global and regional functional parameters as derived from ECG-gated PET with radionuclide angiography,[36,37] contrast-enhanced CT (40) and even magnetic resonance imaging (MRI) (**Fig. 1**).[38–40] It is feasible even with tracers labeled with short half-life isotopes.[41–43] In addition, Knesaurek and colleagues[44] found that for cardiac rubidium Rb 82 PET global functional parameters from PET scanners operating in 2-dimensional and 3-dimensional mode did not differ, thus offering a dose-efficient access to those clinically relevant parameters in modern PET tomographs. Also, a comparison between contractile analyses in a study comparing patients with 2 different PET tracers (N-13 NH3 + O-15 CO and

N-13 NH3 + [18]F FDG) revealed consistent results[41,45] pointing toward the high stability in routine PET imaging.

Clinically more relevant than technical considerations (however necessary to understand both advantages and limitations) is that gated perfusion PET is superior to gated SPECT MPI[46] and also provides incremental prognostic value as shown by Dorbala and colleagues.[47] The same group investigated, also specifically, the value of vasodilator left ventricular ejection fraction reserve in 510 consecutive patients. They found that a reserve of more than +5% had a positive predictive value of only 41% but a negative predictive value of 97% for excluding severe left main/3-vessel disease. Because this analysis can be embedded without prolonging scan time or increasing dose, this seems to be a valuable addition to the clinical workflow.

This kind of analysis is feasible, as—because of the large number of clinical MPI SPECT examinations—a variety of analysis programs exist for the quantitative and functional analysis. Although it may appear straightforward to use in the case of gated PET, some care has to be taken because the spatial resolution (which also is a function of the used isotope/tracer depending on the energy of the emitted positron) and thus partial volume

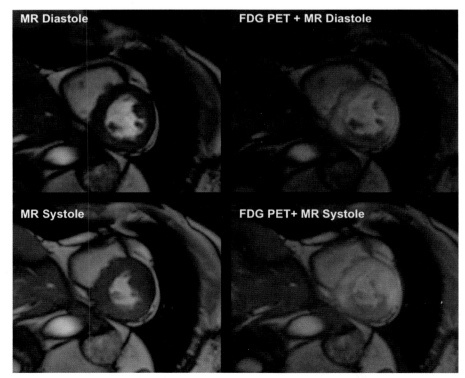

Fig. 1. Simultaneously acquired FDG PET and MRI data from a fully integrated PET/MRI system showing the matching information derived from gated PET and MRI.

effects differ.[48] To establish proper thresholds for rubidium Rb 82 scans, analysis programs were compared[49] and reference values were established.[50] As both studies confirmed—consistent with SPECT MPI[51]—those functional parameters vary significantly between the software programs and therefore cannot be used interchangeably.

As mentioned previously, the assessment of myocardial viability by ^{18}F FDG-PET is a widely used approach to characterize myocardial tissue and identify those viable regions that could benefit from interventions.[7,8] This is typically performed using the static distribution of ^{18}F FDG, but the integration of contractile information is possible as well.[52] In patients with ischemic cardiomyopathy undergoing myocardial viability assessment, incremental prognostic value over viability information alone was found (n = 90).[53] However, in another study, the integration of gated FDG into assessment of myocardial viability without a perfusion scan (n = 38) showed that the incremental value of contractile parameters was not fully conclusive[54,55]; thus, further investigation and larger studies are needed.

The assessment of functional contractile parameters with implanted devices, such as pacemakers or implantable cardioverter-defibrillator (ICD) leads, can be imaged using PET/CT systems[56] as long as proper metal artifact reduction is used for the CT used in the attenuation correction. The fact that cardiac MR imaging in this increasing population is not straightforward makes PET an attractive alternative.

The addition of gated acquisitions to conventional protocols adds relevant prognostic information basically at no cost.

PHASE ANALYSIS

Again with roots reaching back to planar imaging, harmonic phase analysis is also feasible with gated PET studies and gained substantial attention in the last years.[57,58] The phase analysis with gated equilibrium planar nuclear imaging was one of the earliest examples of the use of computers in medical imaging and successfully introduced the use of color displays.[59] Initially applied to the detection, evaluation, and follow-up of left ventricular (LV) regional wall motion abnormalities, this approach was widely and successfully used before cardiac MRI was clinically established. Technically, the signal from the blood pool is analyzed using harmonic (Fourier) analysis and the parameters describing this contraction are calculated. After the extension to gated blood pool SPECT,[60,61] phase analysis migrated many years later to myocardial SPECT

perfusion imaging in which basically the same concept was applied. Here the signal from the myocardial walls was used instead of the blood pool data.[62,63] This technique is based on the fact that the myocardial wall thickens during contraction and—because of the limited spatial resolution of SPECT—the signal from that region increases during systole because of the partial volume effect. This technical development was implemented rapidly in patients before cardiac resynchronization therapy (CRT). This intervention is a well-recognized option for patients with end-stage heart failure. Unfortunately, a subset of patients does not respond to CRT, making a noninvasive, medical imaging–based identification of nonresponders a desirable option.[64] This concept was extensively discussed in a recent review by Henneman and colleagues.[65]

Because SPECT images are basically similar to PET images, the application of phase analysis is straightforward and appeals especially to PET viability imaging. Pazhenkottil and colleagues[66] applied this analysis to ^{18}F FDG data and compared the results with SPECT MPI data from the same patients. They found excellent agreement between the modalities and pointed out that this approach allowed the simultaneous assessment of viability and dyssynchrony in one examination. Another study integrated the positioning of pace maker leads with dyssynchrony analysis by ^{18}F FDG-PET and identified potential reasons for CRT nonresponders, which is again pointing to the valuable role of PET in this field (**Fig. 2**).[67]

Just as in SPECT MPI, PET flow tracers can be used. Another comparison between the 2 methodologies (SPECT and PET) suggested that contractile phase abnormalities were more widespread than regional wall motion abnormalities offering incremental value, which is especially attractive, because no additional measurement, is performed.[68] This concept of examining patients with LV dysfunction showing both abnormal regional contractility and motion (dyssynergy) and altered synchronicity of contraction (asynchrony) was recently adapted to gated PET. Initial studies applied it to rubidium Rb 82 perfusion studies acquired in resting state and, using pharmaceutical stress and derived normal limit,[69] found high sensitivities and specificities (80%/90% for men; 92%/75% for women; *P* value not significant) for the detection of wall motion abnormalities in patients with ECG evidence of a left bundle branch block. Furthermore, the reported normal values did not differ between the previously published values for SPECT MPI studies.[62]

Also using perfusion rubidium Rb 82 studies, Aljaroudi and colleagues[70] investigated the

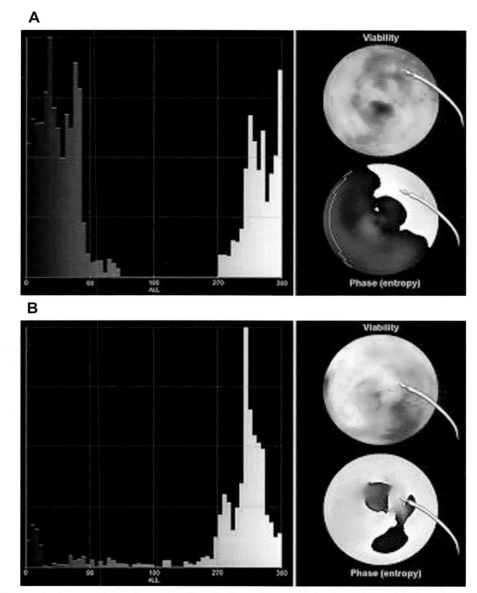

Fig. 2. Harmonic phase analysis of gated PET studies in patients with implanted CRT. (A) Phase histogram (*left*) and polar map (*right*) of LV ^{18}F FDG uptake and global phase entropy (lower polar map) in relation to LV pacemaker lead position in a nonresponder (A) and responder (B) to CRT. Compared with the responder patient, the nonresponder shows a broader bandwidth in the phase histogram and LV lead located in area of nonviable myocardium and high phase entropy. (*Reprinted from* Uebleis C, Ulbrich M, Tegtmeyer R. Electrocardiogram-gated 18F-FDG PET/CT hybrid imaging in patients with unsatisfactory response to cardiac resynchronization therapy: initial clinical results. J Nucl Med 2010;52(1):67–71; with permission from Society of Nuclear Medicine.)

incremental value of LV mechanical dyssynchrony in a large population of almost 500 patients with narrow QRS cardiomyopathy. The investigators were able to show that LV mechanical dyssynchrony is an independent predictor of all-cause mortality with the potential to identify those subjects in whom the survival benefit might differ between medical therapy and bypass surgery.[70] Recently, the same group published an analysis comparing the phase analysis of static rest and dipyridamole stress rubidium Rb 82 studies, which are acquired in the same imaging session. The authors included 91 patients with normal MPI and ejection fraction greater than 55% and 126 patients with and ejection fraction less than 35%. They found that LV mechanical dyssynchrony is smaller when delineated from the stress data in patients with normal MPI without a relation to the LV ejection fraction. As in patients with normal flow tracer distribution patterns (at least in absence of absolute flow quantification) a decision has to be made whether the rest or the stress phase analysis is used, and further validation studies are obviously required. Another relevant technical aspect of this study is worth mentioning: the image data were generated on a conventional, dedicated PET system operating in 2-dimensional mode and a hybrid PET/CT acquiring data in 3-dimensional mode, the latter offering higher sensitivity, which allowed the injected dose to be reduced. However, the absence of septa increases the scatter, which is, especially in perfusion experiments, a potential limitation. Nonetheless, no evidence was found that the different systems affected the results of phase analysis.

IMPROVED IMAGE QUALITY BY INTEGRATING GATED DATA

In addition to extracting functional parameters from gated studies, these acquisitions can also be used to improve image quality. Slomka and colleagues[71] developed a technique called *motion frozen* display for SPECT data. Basically, all gated frames are "warped" to a reference frame, thus increasing the image quality (as in summing all gated images) but avoiding the effects of motion blur while summing. Because of the image similarities between SPECT and PET, this approach was subsequently extended to PET, and images with excellent spatial resolution were produced. This

might be of value in hybrid PET/CT or PET/MR fusion display (**Fig. 3**).[72]

RESPIRATORY GATED PET AND APPLICATIONS OF LIST MODE ACQUISITIONS

Respiratory motion in the thorax results in potential misalignment between PET and CT data. CT images are acquired during very short scan times, whereas a typical PET scan lasts several minutes, thus collecting emission data over several breathing cycles. Therefore, motion-induced inconsistencies arise between emission and transmission, which may result in artifacts after attenuation correction. Respiration-induced effects were studied extensively for oncology imaging. In addition, the combined effects of cardiac contraction and respiratory motion might have to be considered for cardiac imaging.[73] From a technical point of view, respiratory gating is as feasible as cardiac gating in PET imaging. Instead of the ECG circuitry, a detection system for breathing motion is used. In most cases, a pneumatic device is integrated into an elastic belt, which is fastened around the lower chest of the patient. This technique is widely used in MRIs where it represents a standard procedure to limit artifacts from respiration. In addition, it is a very effective approach to monitor patient compliance to breathing instructions, because most cardiac MRI sequences are performed during (end-expiration) breath hold.

Independent of the technical implementation, it is important to remember, that a histogram of human respiratory signal is qualitatively different from that of cardiac gating signal. Breathing patterns can be very irregular and may vary substantially over the duration of a PET acquisition.

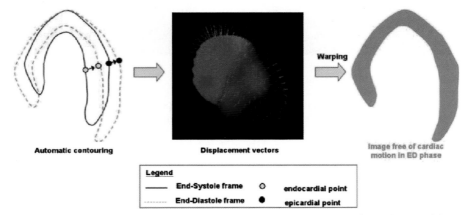

Fig. 3. Principle of the Cardiac Motion Frozen technique to generate an image from the gated frames without motion blur. (*Left*) Motion tracking of the LV. (*Middle*) Displacement vectors between each cardiac phase. (*Right*) Generation of an image that is free of cardiac motion but with the noise of a summed static image. (*Reprinted from* Le Meunier L, Slomka PJ, Dey D, et al. Motion frozen (18)F-FDG cardiac PET. J Nucl Cardiol 2011;18(2):259–66; with permission from Springer Science+BusinessMedia.)

The possibility of arbitrary combinations of histogramming settings yields another advantage for short-lived isotopes such as rubidium Rb 82 or ammonia N 13. In conventional ammonia PET imaging, dynamic data are acquired for about 10 minutes after tracer injection followed by an ECG-gated acquisition for another 10 minutes. Because of the isotope decay, the gated data used to suffer from a reduced signal-to-noise-ratio. In list mode, however, the data after tracer injection can be used to generate dynamic images to quantify absolute blood flow as well. In addition, after focusing on the data immediately after ammonia extraction from the blood (typically after 2–3 minutes for ammonia), any combination of cardiac or respiratory gating can be applied (**Fig. 4**). This method has not been applied clinically yet, but Sayre and colleagues[74] proposed a protocol to efficiently assess both gated and dynamic imaging using rubidium Rb 82.

COMBINING CARDIAC AND RESPIRATORY GATING (DUAL GATING)

The combination of ECG and respiratory gating currently is the domain of research protocols and not commercially available. As shown in **Fig. 4**, in the dual gating example, the number of matching events may vary according to the likelihood of certain combinations over others (eg, the combination of systole and expiration is more likely than systole and inspiration). The trigger phases used in this particular case are indicated as filled (ECG) and open (respiratory) boxes below the trigger traces. Martinez-Möller and colleagues[75] showed that the respiratory motion of the heart had a significant elastic component, which was of the same magnitude as the spatial resolution of current PET cameras; however, overall effects were modest (**Fig. 5**). Also, other groups showed its feasibility, as Teras and colleagues[76] and Gigengack and colleagues[77] demonstrated recently.

From a clinical point of view, the effects of respiratory motion on cardiac diagnosis are yet unknown and need further investigation. However, Teras and colleagues[76] pointed toward the potential for molecular imaging. Hot-spot imaging, for example, of vulnerable plaques in the coronaries,[78] may also profit from complex gating schemes. In such a scenario, small structures might show tracer retention; however, it is blurred by cardiac and respiratory motion.[79] Motion correction schemes based on the trigger signals could recover this tracer signal. It may also be speculated that

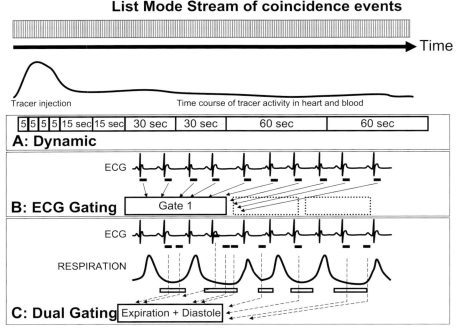

Fig. 4. List mode acquisitions offer the advantage of flexible, retrospective generation of image data according to various sorting criteria. Three histogramming examples using the list mode stream are illustrated. (*A*) Dynamic framing using the full data stream with frame rates adjusted to the kinetics of the tracer. (*B*) Sorting according to the ECG as soon as the tracer reached an equilibrium phase. (*C*) Dual ECG and respiratory gating. In this extension to (*B*), the trigger phases used in the particular example are indicated as filled (ECG) and open (respiratory) boxes when the patient's heart and lungs are both in diastolic phase or end-expiratory state, respectively.

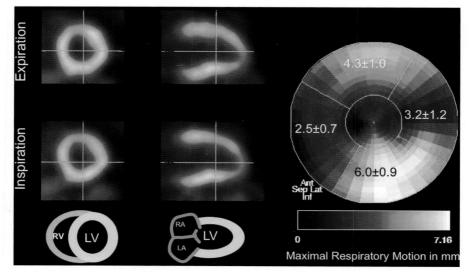

Fig. 5. Ammonia N 13 study summed between 2 and 10 minutes post injection from list mode data that were histogrammed into 6 respiratory and 2 cardiac phases. Images show the end diastolic frame in end-inspiration and end-expiration. The crossed lines in the short and long axis image are spatially fixed to show the motion. In addition, a polar map of the maximal motion differences between the end states is given. (*Reprinted from* Nekolla SG. Dynamic and gated PET: quantitative imaging of the heart revisited. Nuklearmedizin 2005;44(Suppl 1):S41–5; with permission.)

image-derived arterial input functions based on end-respiration/end-diastolic images will improve because spillover from the myocardium is minimized.

SUMMARY

Gated PET was validated in numerous studies over the last decade and showed clear incremental value in both ischemia and viability imaging. Modern PET/CT systems with list mode acquisitions offer powerful and convenient means for dynamic and gated PET imaging in the clinical arena of multimodality imaging. The integration of quantitative, regional, multiparameter information will further enhance the diagnostic quality of PET cardiac imaging.

REFERENCES

1. Schwaiger M, Ziegler S, Nekolla SG. PET/CT: challenge for nuclear cardiology. J Nucl Med 2005; 46(10):1664–78.
2. Schwaiger M, Ziegler SI, Nekolla SG. PET/CT challenge for the non-invasive diagnosis of coronary artery disease. Eur J Radiol 2010;73(3):494–503.
3. Nekolla SG, Reder S, Saraste A, et al. Evaluation of the novel myocardial perfusion positron-emission tomography tracer 18F-BMS-747158-02: comparison to 13N-ammonia and validation with microspheres in a pig model. Circulation 2009;119(17):2333–42.
4. Yu M, Nekolla SG, Schwaiger M, et al. The next generation of cardiac positron emission tomography imaging agents: discovery of flurpiridaz F-18 for detection of coronary disease. Semin Nucl Med 2011;41(4):305–13.
5. Berman DS, Germano G, Slomka PJ. Improvement in PET myocardial perfusion image quality and quantification with flurpiridaz F 18. J Nucl Cardiol 2012;19(Suppl 1):S38–45.
6. Camici PG, Rimoldi OE. The clinical value of myocardial blood flow measurement. J Nucl Med 2009;50(7):1076–87.
7. Schinkel AF, Poldermans D, Elhendy A, et al. Assessment of myocardial viability in patients with heart failure. J Nucl Med 2007;48(7):1135–46.
8. Camici PG, Prasad SK, Rimoldi OE. Stunning, hibernation, and assessment of myocardial viability. Circulation 2008;117(1):103–14.
9. Tillisch J, Brunken R, Marshall R, et al. Reversibility of cardiac wall-motion abnormalities predicted by positron tomography. N Engl J Med 1986;314(14):884–8.
10. Haas F, Haehnel CJ, Picker W, et al. Preoperative positron emission tomographic viability assessment and perioperative and postoperative risk in patients with advanced ischemic heart disease. J Am Coll Cardiol 1997;30(7):1693–700.
11. Dobrucki LW, Sinusas AJ. PET and SPECT in cardiovascular molecular imaging. Nat Rev Cardiol 2010; 7(1):38–47.
12. Gelfand MJ, Thomas SR. Effective use of computers in nuclear medicine. New York: McGraw-Hill; 1988.

13. Borer JS, Bacharach SL, Green MV, et al. Real-time radionuclide cineangiography in the noninvasive evaluation of global and regional left ventricular function at rest and during exercise in patients with coronary-artery disease. N Engl J Med 1977; 296(15):839–44.

14. Bacharach SL, Green MV, Borer JS, et al. ECG-gated scintillation probe measurement of left ventricular function. J Nucl Med 1977;18(12):1176–83.

15. Schwaiger M, Ratib O, Henze E, et al. Limitations of quantitative phase analysis of radionuclide angiograms for detecting coronary artery disease in patients with impaired left ventricular function. Am Heart J 1984;108(4 Pt 1):942–9.

16. Budinger TF, Cahoon JL, Derenzo SE, et al. Three dimensional imaging of the myocardium with radionuclides. Radiology 1977;125(2):433–9.

17. Moore ML, Murphy PH, Burdine JA. ECG-gated emission computed tomography of the cardiac blood pool. Radiology 1980;134(1):233–5.

18. Tamaki N, Mukai T, Ishii Y, et al. Multiaxial tomography of heart chambers by gated blood-pool emission computed tomography using a rotating gamma camera. Radiology 1983;147(2):547–54.

19. Barat JL, Brendel AJ, Colle JP, et al. Quantitative analysis of left-ventricular function using gated single photon emission tomography. J Nucl Med 1984;25(11):1167–74.

20. Okada RD, Boucher CA, Strauss HW, et al. Exercise radionuclide imaging approaches to coronary artery disease. Am J Cardiol 1980;46(7):1188–204.

21. Treves S, Hill TC, VanPraagh R, et al. Computed tomography of the heart using thallium-201 in children. Radiology 1979;132(3):707–10.

22. Kiat H, Maddahi J, Roy LT, et al. Comparison of technetium 99m methoxy isobutyl isonitrile and thallium 201 for evaluation of coronary artery disease by planar and tomographic methods. Am Heart J 1989;117(1):1–11.

23. Huang SC, Hoffman EJ, Phelps ME, et al. Quantitation in positron emission computed tomography: 2. Effects of inaccurate attenuation correction. J Comput Assist Tomogr 1979;3(6):804–14.

24. Martinez-Moller A, Souvatzoglou M, Navab N, et al. Artifacts from misaligned CT in cardiac perfusion PET/CT studies: frequency, effects, and potential solutions. J Nucl Med 2007;48(2):188–93.

25. Gould KL, Pan T, Loghin C, et al. Frequent diagnostic errors in cardiac PET/CT due to misregistration of CT attenuation and emission PET images: a definitive analysis of causes, consequences, and corrections. J Nucl Med 2007;48(7):1112–21.

26. Lautamaki R, Brown TL, Merrill J, et al. CT-based attenuation correction in (82)Rb-myocardial perfusion PET-CT: incidence of misalignment and effect on regional tracer distribution. Eur J Nucl Med Mol Imaging 2008;35(2):305–10.

27. Slomka PJ, Dey D, Duvall WL, et al. Advances in nuclear cardiac instrumentation with a view towards reduced radiation exposure. Curr Cardiol Rep 2012; 14(2):208–16.

28. Hoffman EJ, Phelps ME, Wisenberg G, et al. Electrocardiographic gating in positron emission computed tomography. J Comput Assist Tomogr 1979;3(6): 733–9.

29. Yamashita K, Tamaki N, Yonekura Y, et al. Quantitative analysis of regional wall motion by gated myocardial positron emission tomography: validation and comparison with left ventriculography. J Nucl Med 1989;30(11):1775–86.

30. Miller TR, Wallis JW, Landy BR, et al. Measurement of global and regional left ventricular function by cardiac PET. J Nucl Med 1994;35(6):999–1005.

31. Porenta G, Kuhle W, Sinha S, et al. Parameter estimation of cardiac geometry by ECG-gated PET imaging: validation using magnetic resonance imaging and echocardiography. J Nucl Med 1995;36(6):1123–9.

32. Buvat I, Bartlett ML, Kitsiou AN, et al. A "hybrid" method for measuring myocardial wall thickening from gated PET/SPECT images. J Nucl Med 1997; 38(2):324–9.

33. Humm JL, Rosenfeld A, Del Guerra A. From PET detectors to PET scanners. Eur J Nucl Med Mol Imaging 2003;30(11):1574–97.

34. Erdi YE, Nehmeh SA, Mulnix T, et al. PET performance measurements for an LSO-based combined PET/CT scanner using the National Electrical Manufacturers Association NU 2-2001 standard. J Nucl Med 2004;45(5):813–21.

35. Pichler BJ, Wehrl HF, Judenhofer MS. Latest advances in molecular imaging instrumentation. J Nucl Med 2008;49(Suppl 2):5S–23S.

36. Hattori N, Bengel FM, Mehilli J, et al. Global and regional functional measurements with gated FDG PET in comparison with left ventriculography. Eur J Nucl Med 2001;28(2):221–9.

37. Saab G, Dekemp RA, Ukkonen H, et al. Gated fluorine 18 fluorodeoxyglucose positron emission tomography: determination of global and regional left ventricular function and myocardial tissue characterization. J Nucl Cardiol 2003;10(3):297–303.

38. Schaefer WM, Lipke CS, Nowak B, et al. Validation of QGS and 4D-MSPECT for quantification of left ventricular volumes and ejection fraction from gated 18F-FDG PET: comparison with cardiac MRI. J Nucl Med 2004;45(1):74–9.

39. Schaefer WM, Lipke CS, Nowak B, et al. Validation of an evaluation routine for left ventricular volumes, ejection fraction and wall motion from gated cardiac FDG PET: a comparison with cardiac magnetic resonance imaging. Eur J Nucl Med Mol Imaging 2003; 30(4):545–53.

40. Slart RH, Bax JJ, de Jong RM, et al. Comparison of gated PET with MRI for evaluation of left ventricular

function in patients with coronary artery disease. J Nucl Med 2004;45(2):176–82.

41. Okazawa H, Takahashi M, Hata T, et al. Quantitative evaluation of myocardial blood flow and ejection fraction with a single dose of (13)NH(3) and Gated PET. J Nucl Med 2002;43(8):999–1005.

42. Hickey KT, Sciacca RR, Bokhari S, et al. Assessment of cardiac wall motion and ejection fraction with gated PET using N-13 ammonia. Clin Nucl Med 2004;29(4):243–8.

43. Kanayama S, Matsunari I, Hirayama A, et al. Assessment of global and regional left ventricular function by electrocardiographic gated N-13 ammonia positron emission tomography in patients with coronary artery disease. Circ J 2005;69(2):177–82.

44. Knesaurek K, Machac J, Ho Kim J. Comparison of 2D, 3D high dose and 3D low dose gated myocardial 82Rb PET imaging. BMC Nucl Med 2007;7:4.

45. Khorsand A, Graf S, Eidherr H, et al. Gated cardiac 13N-NH3 PET for assessment of left ventricular volumes, mass, and ejection fraction: comparison with electrocardiography-gated 18F-FDG PET. J Nucl Med 2005;46(12):2009–13.

46. Bateman TM, Heller GV, McGhie AI, et al. Diagnostic accuracy of rest/stress ECG-gated Rb-82 myocardial perfusion PET: comparison with ECG-gated Tc-99m sestamibi SPECT. J Nucl Cardiol 2006;13(1):24–33.

47. Dorbala S, Hachamovitch R, Curillova Z, et al. Incremental prognostic value of gated Rb-82 positron emission tomography myocardial perfusion imaging over clinical variables and rest LVEF. JACC Cardiovasc Imaging 2009;2(7):846–54.

48. Hoffman EJ, Huang SC, Phelps ME. Quantitation in positron emission computed tomography: 1. Effect of object size. J Comput Assist Tomogr 1979;3(3):299–308.

49. Menezes LJ, Groves AM, Prvulovich E, et al. Assessment of left ventricular function at rest using rubidium-82 myocardial perfusion PET: comparison of four software algorithms with simultaneous 64-slice coronary CT angiography. Nucl Med Commun 2009;30(12):918–25.

50. Bravo PE, Chien D, Javadi M, et al. Reference ranges for LVEF and LV volumes from electrocardiographically gated 82Rb cardiac PET/CT using commercially available software. J Nucl Med 2010;51(6):898–905.

51. Knollmann D, Winz OH, Meyer PT, et al. Gated myocardial perfusion SPECT: algorithm-specific influence of reorientation on calculation of left ventricular volumes and ejection fraction. J Nucl Med 2008;49(10):1636–42.

52. Hor G, Kranert WT, Maul FD, et al. Gated metabolic positron emission tomography (GAPET) of the myocardium: 18F-FDG-PET to optimize recognition of myocardial hibernation. Nucl Med Commun 1998;19(6):535–45.

53. Santana CA, Shaw LJ, Garcia EV, et al. Incremental prognostic value of left ventricular function by myocardial ECG-gated FDG PET imaging in patients with ischemic cardiomyopathy. J Nucl Cardiol 2004;11(5):542–50.

54. Slart RH, Bax JJ, van Veldhuisen DJ, et al. Prediction of functional recovery after revascularization in patients with coronary artery disease and left ventricular dysfunction by gated FDG-PET. J Nucl Cardiol 2006;13(2):210–9.

55. Arrighi JA. Assessment of myocardial viability: more than measurements of radiotracer uptake alone. J Nucl Cardiol 2006;13(2):180–3.

56. DiFilippo FP, Brunken RC. Do implanted pacemaker leads and ICD leads cause metal-related artifact in cardiac PET/CT? J Nucl Med 2005;46(3):436–43.

57. Links JM, Douglass KH, Wagner HN Jr. Patterns of ventricular emptying by Fourier analysis of gated blood-pool studies. J Nucl Med 1980;21(10):978–82.

58. Bacharach SL, Green MV, Bonow RO, et al. A method for objective evaluation of functional images. J Nucl Med 1982;23(4):285–90.

59. Deconinck F, Bossuyt A, Hermanne A. A cyclic color scale as an essential requirement in functional imaging of periodic phenomena. Med Phys 1979;6:331.

60. Nakajima K, Taniguchi M, Bunko H, et al. Functional mapping of ventricular contraction and phase using single-photon emission computed tomography (SPECT). Nucl Med Commun 1986;7(11):825–30.

61. Chevalier P, Bontemps L, Fatemi M, et al. Gated blood-pool SPECT evaluation of changes after radiofrequency catheter ablation of accessory pathways: evidence for persistent ventricular preexcitation despite successful therapy. J Am Coll Cardiol 1999;34(6):1839–46.

62. Chen J, Garcia EV, Folks RD, et al. Onset of left ventricular mechanical contraction as determined by phase analysis of ECG-gated myocardial perfusion SPECT imaging: development of a diagnostic tool for assessment of cardiac mechanical dyssynchrony. J Nucl Cardiol 2005;12(6):687–95.

63. Chen J, Henneman MM, Trimble MA, et al. Assessment of left ventricular mechanical dyssynchrony by phase analysis of ECG-gated SPECT myocardial perfusion imaging. J Nucl Cardiol 2008;15(1):127–36.

64. Henneman MM, Chen J, Dibbets-Schneider P, et al. Can LV dyssynchrony as assessed with phase analysis on gated myocardial perfusion SPECT predict response to CRT? J Nucl Med 2007;48(7):1104–11.

65. Henneman MM, van der Wall EE, Ypenburg C, et al. Nuclear imaging in cardiac resynchronization therapy. J Nucl Med 2007;48(12):2001–10.

66. Pazhenkottil AP, Buechel RR, Nkoulou R, et al. Left ventricular dyssynchrony assessment by phase analysis from gated PET-FDG scans. J Nucl Cardiol 2011;18(5):920–5.

67. Uebleis C, Ulbrich M, Tegtmeyer R, et al. Electrocardiogram-gated 18F-FDG PET/CT hybrid imaging in patients with unsatisfactory response to cardiac resynchronization therapy: initial clinical results. J Nucl Med 2011;52(1):67–71.

68. Nichols KJ, Van Tosh A, Wang Y, et al. Relationships between blood pool and myocardial perfusion-gated SPECT global and regional left ventricular function measurements. Nucl Med Commun 2009; 30(4):292–9.

69. Cooke CD, Esteves FP, Chen J, et al. Left ventricular mechanical synchrony from stress and rest 82Rb PET myocardial perfusion ECG-gated studies: differentiating normal from LBBB patients. J Nucl Cardiol 2011;18(6):1076–85.

70. Aljaroudi W, Alraies MC, Hachamovitch R, et al. Association of left ventricular mechanical dyssynchrony with survival benefit from revascularization: a study of gated positron emission tomography in patients with ischemic LV dysfunction and narrow QRS. Eur J Nucl Med Mol Imaging 2012;39:1581–91.

71. Slomka PJ, Nishina H, Berman DS, et al. "Motion-frozen" display and quantification of myocardial perfusion. J Nucl Med 2004;45(7):1128–34.

72. Le Meunier L, Slomka PJ, Dey D, et al. Motion frozen (18)F-FDG cardiac PET. J Nucl Cardiol 2011;18(2): 259–66.

73. Livieratos L, Rajappan K, Stegger L, et al. Respiratory gating of cardiac PET data in list-mode acquisition. Eur J Nucl Med Mol Imaging 2006;33(5):584–8.

74. Sayre GA, Bacharach SL, Dae MW, et al. Combining dynamic and ECG-gated (8)(2)Rb-PET for practical implementation in the clinic. Nucl Med Commun 2012;33(1):4–13.

75. Martinez-Möller A, Zikic D, Botnar RM, et al. Dual cardiac-respiratory gated PET: implementation and results from a feasibility study. Eur J Nucl Med Mol Imaging 2007;34(9):1447–54.

76. Teras M, Kokki T, Durand-Schaefer N, et al. Dual-gated cardiac PET-clinical feasibility study. Eur J Nucl Med Mol Imaging 2010;37(3):505–16.

77. Gigengack F, Ruthotto L, Burger M, et al. Motion correction in dual gated cardiac PET using mass-preserving image registration. IEEE Trans Med Imaging 2012;31(3):698–712.

78. Cheng VY, Slomka PJ, Le Meunier L, et al. Coronary arterial 18F-FDG uptake by fusion of PET and coronary CT angiography at sites of percutaneous stenting for acute myocardial infarction and stable coronary artery disease. J Nucl Med 2012;53(4): 575–83.

79. Delso G, Martinez-Möller A, Bundschuh RA, et al. Preliminary study of the detectability of coronary plaque with PET. Phys Med Biol 2011;56(7):2145–60.

Four-Dimensional PET-CT in Radiation Oncology

Osama R. Mawlawi, PhD[a],*, Laurence E. Court, PhD[b]

KEYWORDS

- 4D PET-CT • Treatment planning • Radiotherapy • Gross tumor volume • Response assessment

KEY POINTS

- Radiation therapy is at a point at which accurate delineation of the tumor is critical and identification of subvolumes that may be treatment-resistant can be accurately planned and treated. Four-dimensional (4D) PET-CT facilitates this for tumors affected by respiratory motion.
- Although this is still a research topic, the tools and techniques are in place for practical clinical implementation over the next few years.
- There is increasing evidence that PET can play an important part in predicting and assessing dose response for both tumors and normal tissues. The introduction of 4D PET can potentially improve the quality of this data.

INTRODUCTION: BUILDING THE ENVIRONMENT FOR FOUR-DIMENSIONAL PET-CT IN RADIATION ONCOLOGY

The goal of radiation therapy (RT) is to kill cancerous cells while minimizing damage to nearby normal tissues. Thus, it is important to conform the radiation dose to a specific volume that includes the region of known disease (eg, disease visible on a CT image) and regions of suspected subclinical, microscopic, malignant disease that may not be visible. These volumes are known as the gross target volume (GTV) and clinical target volume (CTV), respectively[1,2] (**Fig. 1**). In the presence of respiratory motion, the treated volume must be further increased to ensure that the target is adequately covered. This concept is known as the internal target volume (ITV).[2] It is defined as the volume that encompasses all positions of the target volume (CTV) when all respiratory phases are considered (**Fig. 2**), although other approaches have been investigated.[3–5] For most lung tumors the peak-to-peak respiratory motion is less than 1 cm, but motion of 2 cm or more can be found,

and is more likely for targets close to the diaphragm, including the liver and kidneys.[6,7] Finally, an additional expansion of the target volume (2–10 mm in all directions, depending on the treatment site and patient treatment technique) is made to account for geometric uncertainties such as variations in patient setup from day to day. This final volume is known as the planning target volume (PTV).[2] Each of these volume expansion results in an increase in the amount of normal tissue that is being irradiated. Thus, although only the GTV and CTV are treated, to account for organ motion and other uncertainties it is necessary to increase the treatment volume by several cubic centimeters. Given the magnitude of these uncertainties faced during RT treatment planning and delivery, until fairly recently there was not a strong push for the increased accuracy (geometric and absolute standardized uptake value [SUV]) possible with four-dimensional (4D) PET compared with three-dimensional (3D) PET.

However, over the last decade these issues have been progressively addressed by the clinical introduction of various treatment and imaging

[a] Department of Imaging Physics, The University of Texas MD Anderson Cancer Center, 1515 Holcombe Boulevard Unit 1352, Houston, TX 77030, USA; [b] Department of Radiation Physics, The University of Texas MD Anderson Cancer Center, 1515 Holcombe Boulevard Unit 94, Houston, TX 77030, USA
* Corresponding author.
E-mail address: OMawlawi@mdanderson.org

PET Clin 8 (2013) 81–94
http://dx.doi.org/10.1016/j.cpet.2012.09.010
1556-8598/13/$ – see front matter © 2013 Elsevier Inc. All rights reserved.

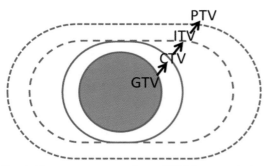

Fig. 1. The gross tumor volume (GTV) is expanded to account for subclinical disease, motion, and setup and other uncertainties, giving the clinical target volume (CTV), internal target volume (ITV), and planning target volume (PTV), respectively.

technologies in radiation oncology, including intensity modulated RT (IMRT) treatment techniques, 4D CT imaging capabilities, image-guided RT (IGRT) patient setup techniques, and respiratory motion management techniques. These techniques are now widely available and most are considered standard-of-care in RT. Their progressive introduction and acceptance by the radiation oncology community was a necessary precursor to the need for 4D PET, the subject of this article, each briefly summarized below.

IMRT,[8,9] and its recent variation volumetric modulated arc therapy[10,11] allows for the delivery of extremely complicated dose distributions that

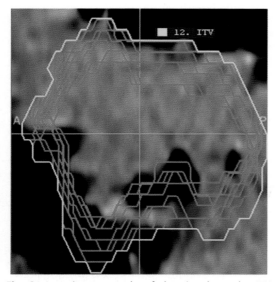

Fig. 2. A patient example of showing how the ITV (*yellow outer-envelope*) is created by the Boolean sum of the individual GTVs from each respiratory phase (*purple lines*). This volume would be further expanded to give the CTV and PTV. (*Courtesy of N. Yakoumakis.*)

closely conform to the target volume (PTV), and can be shaped to avoid adjacent critical structures. The excellent conformality achievable with these techniques emphasizes the need to accurately define the target itself. These techniques also facilitate the use of dose painting, in which different regions of the target are irradiated to different dose levels. Historically this was achieved by treating the entire volume to a certain dose, then shrinking the treatment volume to give a higher dose to regions of higher risk (ie, the GTV). Dose painting allows multiple dose levels to be treated simultaneously. This is the basis of the use of PET data for dose painting (**Fig. 3**; see later discussion).

The introduction of IGRT has improved the geometric accuracy of RT treatments. There are many different approaches,[12–14] but the most common one uses x-ray tubes and detectors which are attached to the medical linear accelerator such that orthogonal x-ray images or cone-beam CT images can be taken of the patient immediately before irradiation. These images are compared with the CT images used for the treatment plan and the patient position is then adjusted. The residual positioning uncertainty after the use of IGRT can be a few millimeters or less, meaning that the radiation dose is delivered in a highly conformal manner day after day, potentially allowing for a reduction in the PTV margins. Again, this development in treatment technology emphasizes the need to accurately define the target. As margins are reduced, the uncertainties in target definition can result in a geometric miss of the tumor, thus degrading the likelihood of successful treatment.

Historically, respiratory motion was accounted for by either adding a fixed margin, based on population data, or by determining the treatment aperture based on fluoroscopic imaging. The introduction of 4D CT, the use of which is now standard-of-care in many centers, has greatly improved our ability to understand, and account for, respiratory motion on a patient-specific basis.[15–17] In 4D CT, the patient's respiratory motion is monitored, usually based on external chest motion, and a series of 3D datasets, each representing a different phase of the respiratory cycle is reconstructed. Details of the different approaches to creating this 4D CT dataset are beyond the scope of this article.[16,18,19] By using these datasets to delineate the target it is possible to accurately account for motion and deformations in the target throughout the respiratory cycle. This may allow more accurate patient-specific treatment volumes, perhaps allowing a reduction in ITV margins.[18]

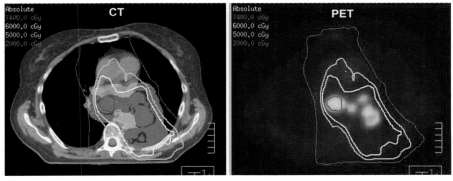

Fig. 3. PET image-guided dose painting. The region with SUV greater than 13.8 is treated to 74 Gy using IMRT, keeping the rest of the target volume to 60 Gy, thus minimizing dose to the normal lung. Here the isodoses (*solid lines*) are superimposed on the CT with target regions identified (*colored volumes*) and on the PET where SUV is shown. (*Reprinted from* Chang JY, Cox JD. Improving radiation conformality in the treatment of non-small cell lung cancer. Semin Radiat Oncol 2010;20(3):171–7; with permission.)

During the last decade, there has been much research into managing the impact of respiratory motion in radiation oncology, thus potentially reducing the ITV expansion and minimizing dose to nearby normal tissues. Although the most common approach is still to include the entire target motion within the treatment volume (as described previously), there are several alternative approaches that can be used, especially for cases in which the respiratory motion would be relatively large. These approaches can be considered in four categories[16]: (1) respiratory-gating techniques in which the radiation beam is administered during a particular phase of the respiratory cycle (eg, either inhale or exhale), (2) breath-hold techniques, (3) forced shallow-breathing techniques, and (4) tumor tracking techniques. The optimal use of an appropriate motion management technique can potentially reduce (or account for) respiratory motion such that the residual motion is less than a few millimeters.[16,20] However, there are many clinical factors that can make this difficult.[16,21] Many of these techniques take advantage of 4D CT techniques for delineating the tumor. For example, if treating with respiratory gating, the target will be delineated only on the respiratory phases for which the radiation beams will be turned on. In addition to allowing reductions in the treatment volume (ITV), because respiratory motion has the effect of blurring the delivered dose distribution,[22] the delivered dose distribution will also be closer to the planned dose distribution than will those without the use of motion management techniques. This reduces one of the barriers to meaningful implementation of SUV-based dose-painting techniques described later.

In summary, the introduction of IMRT, IGRT, 4D CT, and advanced respiratory motion management has made the RT environment ripe for the introduction of 4D PET. Geometric and dosimetric uncertainties have been reduced to a point at which the accurate definition of the target volume is of critical importance, and the use of dose-painting based on biologic information (eg, from PET) can be achieved without significant loss of integrity due to blurring. In addition, there are several other advances in RT treatments[23] that promote this drive to highly accurate treatments,[23] including stereotactic body RT (SBRT), adaptive RT, and particle therapy (eg, protons) that will likely become active users of 4D PET as it becomes more widely used in RT.

PET FOR RT PLANNING

The advent of advanced RT techniques, such as IMRT and ion/proton therapy, which allow for highly conformal target dose distribution, requires careful determination of the gross tumor volume. In this regard, other imaging techniques beyond those that provide structural-anatomic information (CT and MRI) have been proposed to aid in the process of target definition and treatment planning. Functional imaging such as PET, and its more recent variant PET in combination with CT (PET-CT), is one such alternative that has gained wide acceptance. With PET imaging, information about the underlying biologic-biochemical processes can be leveraged to improve the delineation of the GTV and treatment plan. Clearly, the usefulness of the biologic-biochemical signal depends on the radiopharmaceutical used in PET imaging to evaluate and characterize the tumor. Some of the most widely used radiopharmaceuticals are those that can depict glucose metabolism, cell proliferation, and hypoxia.

A large number of studies have shown that PET imaging affect tumor visualization and GTV determination.[24–34] Most studies pertain to lung cancer with particular emphasis on non-small cell lung cancer (NSCLC), whereas head and neck and lymphoma represent a distant second and third, respectively.[35] PET affects GTV determination and RT planning primarily through its superior ability at revealing targets that are not well visualized by other imaging techniques such as CT and MR. These additional targets might be remote to the primary tumor such as in an unsuspected involvement of a lymph node or distant metastasis, or a satellite involvement adjacent to the primary tumor. In addition, PET can impact GTV determination and RT planning by improving the discrimination of equivocal findings on CT/MR images. For example PET has been shown to be able to clearly differentiate between tumor and atelectasis[36,37] or to identify a benign reactive lymphadenopathy (**Fig. 4**). Simply stated, it is much easier for physicians to visualize a tumor clearly when using PET imaging. The clearer visualization of tumors using PET imaging also helps in reducing observer contouring variability while determining the GTV.[38–40]

The incorporation of PET imaging in RT panning can influence the GTV determination in two ways. It can either increase it or decrease it depending on the treatment regimen followed at various centers. For example, the inclusion of previously undetected regional nodal involvement will significantly increase the GTV,[41] whereas the exclusion of enlarged but PET-negative lymph nodes or atelectasis will significantly reduce the GTV.[42] The

recently published Radiation Therapy Oncology Group (RTOG) 0515 study[43] on NSCLC, in which elective nodal irradiation was not used, showed that the GTV was statistically significantly smaller (86.2 mL vs 98.7 mL; $P<.0001$) when using PET-CT for GTV determination compared with CT alone.[44] Whether the GTV is increased or decreased shows the incorporation of PET imaging results in profound changes in RT planning. A recent review article by MacManus and colleagues,[24] which compiled the results of several studies (with >20 subjects) on the impact of PET and PET-CT on RT planning in NSCLC, reported that at least 38% of patients had a change in GTV when PET imaging was used. Other studies involving head and neck cancer have demonstrated similar results.[45–48]

The improvement in RT planning through the incorporation of PET-CT information requires rigorous, consistent, and reproducible PET-CT imaging protocols. This will ensure that the resultant PET-CT images are of the highest quality and, hence, aid in the RT planning process. Standardized oncology PET-CT imaging protocols have been published by several bodies, such as the Society of Nuclear Medicine and Molecular Imaging and the European Association of Nuclear Medicine and Molecular Imaging.[49,50] These protocols, however, need to be modified to specifically account for RT applications. Regardless of the applications, PET imaging should be performed with careful consideration of the amount of injected dose, scan time postinjection, blood

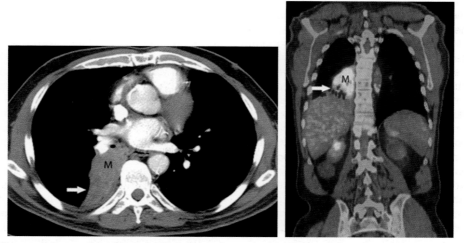

Fig. 4. A 73-year-old man with NSCLC. (*Left*) Chest CT shows a central right lower lobe mass (M) that occludes the right lower lobe bronchus. There is obstructive atelectasis of the right lower lobe distal to the mass (*arrow*). Note that clear differentiation of the mass from atelectatic lung is difficult. (*Right*) Coronal FDG PET-CT shows an FDG-avid mass (M) with distal obstructive atelectasis (*arrow*). Note improved differentiation of malignancy from atelectatic lung can be useful in radiation treatment planning.

glucose level in case of fluorodeoxyGlucose (FDG) imaging and patient comfort. In addition, PET image acquisition and generation parameters should be consistent. Quality assurance and control procedures should be followed to ensure proper scanner calibration, normalization, and alignment between the PET and CT subsystems. For RT planning purposes, accurate positioning to duplicate the treatment position is essential. Ideally, patients should be positioned on a flat table top with all necessary immobilization devices, using the guidance of external lasers and fiducial markers to reproduce the treatment position.[4] Similarly, if training is used to achieve a regular and reproducible breathing pattern, the treatment planning PET-CT study should be consistent with that used for the 4D CT and subsequent treatments.[51]

Several approaches have been suggested with regard to defining the GTV using PET imaging. These techniques range from manual definition using visual assessment to automated techniques using varying approaches that rely on the semi-quantitative nature of PET images.[52] However, none of these techniques has gained exclusivity for PET GTV determination. This is primarily because of the wide variation in their GTV measurements, as well as the lack of a realistic gold standard with which to compare their performance. Ideally, the successful lesion delineation (segmentation) approach should be able to depict the actual spatial and temporal radiotracer distribution on PET images. Moreover, the corresponding PET signal intensity within the segmented lesion should reflect the magnitude of the underlying biologic process. However, even if that is achieved, the segmented lesion might not, in every case, contain all the information needed to define an accurate GTV.[53] For example, in situations of PET false negative, reliance on PET segmented GTVs only will lead to geographic misses. Furthermore, the radiotracer accumulation in different regions, which is the essence of PET imaging, might be confounded by other common biologic processes, such as inflammation, that should not be included in the segmented GTV. At best, PET GTV determination should be used as a starting point for further modification by human intervention. Importantly, the stated improvement of PET imaging on GTV determination and treatment planning previously discussed is not due to the use of PET imaging only but, instead, to the combined use of PET and CT. For example it has been demonstrated that accurate coregistration of PET and CT can decrease the variability in GTV determination compared with the visual analysis of individual PET and CT images shown side by side.[54]

One of the complicating factors that affects PET GTV definition is the limited resolution of PET imaging. Although CT and MRI are characterized by image resolutions on the order of 1 mm, PET imaging has a resolution on the order of 5 to 10 mm. The limited resolution results in the inability to accurately identify tumor boundaries. In this regard, sharp edges appear blurred. In addition, the limited resolution of PET images also results in partial volume effects (PVE) whereby lesions that are smaller than 2 to 3 times the scanner resolution will exhibit a reduction in signal intensity, which could potentially lead to a loss of detectability and an increase in the rate of false negatives. Furthermore, the accumulation of radiopharmaceutical in the background or neighboring region to the tumor results in spill in effects, which further complicates the demarcation of the tumor boundaries on PET images.[55]

One approach to overcome these limitations while leveraging the advantages of using PET imaging for GTV determination is the development of rules and guidelines that are strictly applied when using visual assessment for PET GTV determination. Reports from groups using such an approach have shown that, at least for NSCLC, the consistent use of these guidelines can lead to reproducible RT plans.[56] Other approaches have directly relied on using automated or semiautomated computerized techniques for determining the PET GTV. These approaches usually depend on the PET signal intensity or the SUV as a means to segment the GTV. Segmentations based on such approaches have the potential advantage of consistently generating the same GTV independent of the user, thereby further reducing observer variability while improving reproducibility.

Semiautomated and automated PET GTV segmentation techniques range from the simple to more sophisticated approaches and can be divided into five general groups:

1. Fixed and adaptive threshold techniques
2. Gradient-based techniques
3. Region growing techniques
4. Statistical techniques
5. Learning and texture-based techniques.

Most published papers on PET GTV relate to the first few categories primarily owing to the ease of use of these techniques, particularly in a clinical setting. Furthermore, most manufacturers of RT planning systems have incorporated a few of these simple approaches into their software, further allowing the use of these approaches over other segmentation techniques. A detailed description of all of these techniques is beyond the scope of this article. For a review on this topic, please refer to the article by Zaidi and El Naqa.[52] Each of the segmentation techniques, however, have advantages and shortcomings (see previous discussion) and none have emerged as the preferred approach for PET GTV determination. In addition, new approaches are constantly being introduced. This is an area of active research and is currently the focus of an American Association of Physicists in Medicine (AAPM) task group (TG211).

One recent approach in PET imaging is the incorporation of a point spread function (PSF) during image reconstruction. Such an approach has been demonstrated to potentially recover the PET limited resolution and, hence, reduce PVE. With PSF reconstruction, the PET signal intensity in small tumors can be recovered and the nonstationary resolution profile across the PET scanner field of view will be minimized. It can be conceived that PET GTV segmentation techniques can then be applied following PVE correction or during the PVE correction process.[57,58] Much research is currently ongoing in this area with the potential ability to more accurately identify the tumor boundaries on PET images and, hence, improve PET GTV determination.

4D PET-CT

The main objective of RT planning is to deliver a tumoricidal dose to the target while sparing normal tissue. This objective necessitates the target location to be known at all times for optimal dose delivery. Unfortunately, this situation is not met particularly when treating mobile targets, such as tumors, influenced by respiratory motion. To address this issue, 4D CT techniques (see previous discussion) have been developed. With 4D CT, the tumor extent, as well as motion trajectory and position, can be determined. This information has been shown to help in reducing treatment margins because the expansion of the CTV to PTV is based on patient-specific, instead of population-average, values.[18,59] In a similar manner, 4D PET imaging has been suggested to aid in the process of RT planning. The idea is that 4D PET-CT can have added advantage over 4D CT similar to that of combining PET with CT for GTV determination over CT alone.

The aim of 4D PET, similar to 4D CT, is to minimize motion blur of the resultant images. 4D PET data can be acquired in prospective or retrospective mode. In either case, the acquired PET data are divided into multiple bins each representing a segment of the motion (breathing) cycle. Increasing the number of bins reduces the amount of motion blur per bin but at the cost of increasing image noise. Usually 10 bins are used although several studies have shown that the optimal number of bins depends on the attributes of the motion (breathing) cycle with 6 to 8 bins being suitable for clinical studies.[60–62] PET data binning can be performed using phase (time) or amplitude techniques. Data from each bin are then reconstructed to generate a PET image set corresponding to that segment of the motion cycle. Accurate PET image reconstruction requires an attenuation map that is acquired at the same phase or amplitude (synchronized). 4D CT images that are matched with the bins of the 4D PET data can provide the information to produce 4D PET-CT images. These images can then be used to aid in the RT planning process. Currently, most manufacturers of PET-CT systems have the ability to generate 4D PET-CT images. These manufacturers use similar approaches to synchronize the CT and PET data with the breathing cycle. They also have similar devices to track and record the breathing cycle.[63] This topic is described in detail by Dr Bettinardi and colleagues elsewhere in this issue.

Advantages of 4D PET over nongated PET include greater clarity, ability to improve the delineation of target boundaries, and recovery of PET signal underestimation due to target motion (**Fig. 5**). These advantages, in turn, have the potential of improving the measurement of tumor volume as well as lesion segmentation for GTV determination. Several studies have shown that when using 4D PET, the full extent of lesion volumes is better revealed and the corresponding SUV measurements are increased.[64] These findings suggest that 4D PET can play a role in improving RT planning. More studies, however, are needed to support this suggestion, in particular comparison of the impact of 4D versus nongated PET on RT planning. Currently, most (if not all) RT planning is performed using 4D CT in combination with nongated PET imaging.

Although 4D PET-CT has the ability to reduce motion blur, the resultant PET images are characterized by a low signal to noise (SNR). This is primarily due to the reduced number of events per bin compared with data acquired in nongated mode. As previously mentioned, increasing the number of bins reduces the motion blur per bin but at the cost of increasing image noise and, hence, reducing SNR and image quality. The reduction in SNR and image quality could potentially affect the use of 4D PET data for RT planning and GTV determination. For example, automated tumor segmentation techniques that rely on PET signal intensity could all be affected by the high noise content in the 4D PET images, thereby resulting in a biased GTV. Furthermore, any potential mismatch between the 4D PET and the 4D CT, such as irregularities in breathing between the 4D

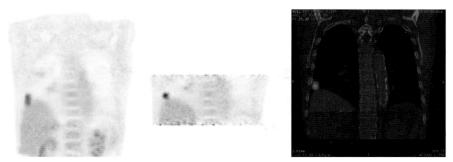

Fig. 5. Coronal PET images of a 77-year-old patient with lung cancer showing a nodule in the lower right lobe. (*Left*) 3D PET data showing smearing of the lesion due to respiratory motion. (*Middle*) 4D PET data suppresses the motion blur, making the tumor more conspicuous while increasing its SUV measurement from 5.0 (nongated PET) to 8.5 (4D PET), (*Right*) 4D PET-CT data showing one of the 4D PET bins (*color*) superimposed on the CT image.

CT and 4D PET data acquisitions, can also affect the PET signal intensity in the target region, which ultimately will bias the GTV determination.

Several techniques have been proposed to address these issues. In the case of low SNR, techniques to combine the PET data following realignment, thereby improving SNR, have been proposed. The realignment can be done following image reconstruction,[65] or during image reconstruction.[66,67] Other approaches of increasing the overall scan time in an effort to increase the detected events per bin have also been proposed. These techniques, however, should be counterbalanced by the knowledge of increase in overall patient movement with increased scanning time. Techniques to minimize irregularities in breathing cycle have also been proposed. These techniques primarily use retrospective binning of PET data acquired in LIST mode. Essentially the LIST PET data are truncated whenever breathing irregularities are encountered. This process is facilitated by synchronizing the breathing trace with the PET data acquisition. Segments of LIST mode PET data that correspond to irregular breathing are then truncated from the PET data before rebinning and reconstruction.[68]

A second potential advantage of using 4D PET imaging for RT planning is the use of the PET signal intensity as a means for boosting the radiation dose to subvolumes within the treatment field. This concept is known as dose painting. The idea of using differential dosing to a tumor based on the biologic signal derived from PET images has its clinical appeal primarily because the main objective of treatment planning is to deliver a tumoricidal dose to the target while sparing normal tissues. Target motion presents a barrier to this objective because the PET signal intensity is artificially underestimated due to motion blur. 4D PET imaging, with its ability to reduce motion blur and

recover the signal intensity, has the potential to take full advantage of this concept.

Two implementations of dose painting have been recognized: dose painting by contours (DPBC) and dose painting by numbers (DPBN). Both of these techniques are currently undergoing extensive investigation and evaluation at several centers.[69–75]

In DPBC, a homogeneous but higher dose is applied to the component of the PTV that was determined from PET image. This can be achieved by either prescribing an additional dose to the PET subvolume of the PTV[23,76] (see **Fig. 3**) or by redistributing the dose of the PTV such that a higher percentage is given to the PET subvolume while keeping the dose to the overall PTV constant.[77] In DPBN, the dose shaping is further refined according to the voxel intensities within the PET subvolume of the PTV,[34,78–80] which is then realized through the application of a mathematical prescription function.[81]

In either case, careful consideration for the PET imaging protocol should be applied to ensure spatial and temporal stability and reproducibility of the PET signal. This issue becomes even more critical when using 4D PET imaging because of its characteristically low SNR, which affects the accuracy of the target SUV measurements. Several studies have shown that the F-18 FDG PET signal intensity changes with scan time postinjection. Furthermore, the quality of the measured PET signal is a direct reflection of the kinetics of the radiopharmaceutical under investigation. For example, in tracers in which active transport is the mechanism of regional uptake such as in the case of FDG, the PET signal will steadily accumulate in tissue until reaching equilibrium. In contrast, hypoxia tracers are diffusion-dependent and, hence, result in a relatively low SNR, therefore placing further restrictions on the imaging protocols. Finally, the issue of how much higher a dose should be applied to these subvolumes is still under investigation. Currently no recommendations are available with only few centers reporting on clinical dose painting studies.[73,75]

A third advantage of 4D PET-CT is the possibility not only looking at biologic structure within the tumor but also how that structure behaves under the influence of motion, something that standard nongated PET cannot show. For example, a moving target might change its shape during its trajectory, thereby necessitating modification of the RT plan, depending on the location of the target, to achieve the desired dose. A recent paper by Aristophanous and colleagues[82] revealed a complex relationship between the various characteristics of the boost regions and the overall target. The investigators concluded that, in cases in which advanced treatment techniques are applied, such as in DP, a close examination of the 4D PET scan should be performed.

Finally, 4D PET-CT supports the notion of gated RT or tracked RT in which the radiation treatment beam either is turned on only during a particular phase of the breathing cycle or is constantly on while tracking the target lesion. In either case, the treatment volumes will be much smaller which potentially can further reduce normal tissue radiation toxicity.

There are several issues that still need to be worked out before 4D PET-CT can be safely and routinely incorporated in treatment planning. Prominent among these issues is the poor resolution and quality of PET images. Current developments of resolution recovery, depth-of-interaction PET,[83] advanced image processing,[84] and time-of-flight PET,[85] carry the promise of improving the resultant PET image quality and bringing 4D PET-CT closer to wider acceptance.

DOSE RESPONSE

In addition to tumor definition and treatment planning using dose painting, PET offers some exciting possibilities that may allow development of a much better understanding of the dose response of tumors and normal tissues. 4D PET is such a new development in radiation oncology that there is minimal published literature on specifically how 4D PET (instead of nongated PET) will allow new advances in dose-response studies. However, these studies typically make use of the SUV that, for targets which are moving because of respiration, can be less reliable when 4D PET is not used. The following is a summary of a few of the published results related to the use of PET to study dose response in the thorax, with the anticipation that, if the investigators did not use 4D PET, then the future use of 4D PET would further improve the robustness of their results. For the purpose of this article, dose response is categorized as prediction versus assessment (ie, using pretreatment or posttreatment scans) and tumor response vs normal tissue response.

Prediction of Treatment Outcome (Tumor)

Pretreatment PET-CT of patients with NSCLC has been shown to be useful in predicting treatment outcome. Specifically, Clarke and colleagues[86] showed that pretreatment maximum SUV (SUV-max) correlated with distant failure for subjects treated with SBRT. Given that SUVmax has been shown to be degraded by respiratory motion, it seems reasonable to postulate that the correlation would have been further improved if 4D PET-CT had been used for this study. Separately, Takeda and colleagues[87] showed that SUVmax in pretreatment images is a predictor for local recurrence for subjects with localized NSCLC after SBRT. Again, the investigators did not use 4D PET, so the measured SUVmax will have been somewhat dependent on the local motion of the tumor; the use of 4D PET may improve the predictive power of SUVmax. This result of Takeda and colleagues[87] is significant because it indicates that a high SUVmax may indicate the use of dose escalation to improve local control. Aerts and colleagues[88] compared pretreatment and posttreatment PET images of NSCLC tumors, and found that the location of residual metabolically active areas remaining in the tumor after therapy corresponded with areas of high SUV in the pretreatment scans, indicating that the pretreatment scan can be used to identify the areas likely to have residual metabolically active areas posttreatment, supporting the use of SUV-based dose painting.

Prediction of Treatment Outcome (Normal Tissue)

Petit and colleagues[89] recently examined the use of PET uptake patterns in lung to identify regions of the lung that are more susceptible to radiation-induced toxicity. They found that the risk of radiation-induced pneumonitis was increased when regions of the lung that had elevated SUV uptake before treatment were included in the irradiated volume. Specifically, they found that the risk increased as the percentage of the fraction of the 5%, 10%, and 20% highest SUV regions that received more than 2 to 5 Gy increased. Although scatter, decay, and attenuation in the PET scans were corrected using the midventilation CT phase, the PET scans themselves were nongated. Because, in this study, the regions of elevated uptake were fairly large, the impact of respiratory motion on the SUV values can be expected to be relatively small, although 4D PET may have been useful here.

De Ruysscher and colleagues[90] examined FDG-PET-CT scans taken on days 0, 7, and 14 after starting RT in patients with NSCLC and found that the maximum SUV in the lung (outside the GTV) increased significantly in the first 2 weeks of treatment, more for patients who developed radiation-induced pneumonitis than for patients who did not develop pneumonitis. McCloskey and colleagues[91] recently reported preliminary data showing that 4D PET-CT taken at time points during the course of RT can provide early indication of esophagitis before it is clinically evident. In extreme cases, esophagitis can result in hospitalization or treatment breaks.[92] The early detection of esophagitis could, potentially, allow for a replan of the treatment to reduce dose to the esophagus. Because the esophagus is subject to respiratory motion[93] the investigators' use of 4D CT may have played an important part in their ability to detect esophagitis at such an early stage. Using the same dataset, the investigators also showed preliminary data that 4D PET could provide an early indicator of radiation-induced pneumonitis.

Assessment of Treatment Response (Tumor)

Treatment response is often quantified using changes in tumor dimensions, as seen in CT images.[94] Although PET scans can also play an important part of the follow-up for many patients,[95,96] PET imaging allows the incorporation of biologic information, such as glucose metabolism,[95] into the assessment of treatment response. Several groups have published studies showing that PET response is significantly correlated with survival.[96,97] Aristophanous and colleagues[98] specifically demonstrated the use of gated PET scans to evaluate treatment-related changes in FDG uptake and compared these results with 3D PET. They showed that the differences in percent of treatment-related SUV change could be larger than 10%, which could result in different response evaluation if using an SUV-based scale to classify the response (eg, the PET Response Criteria in Solid Tumors [PERCIST] criteria[99] or European Organization for Research and Treatment of Cancer [EORTC] recommendations[100]). Thus, PET has an important role in assessing the response of tumors to RT, and the additional accuracy available with 4D PET will further increase its usefulness.

Assessment of Treatment Response (Normal Tissues)

RT of tumors in the lung results in clinically significant symptomatic radiation pneumonitis in 5% to 50% of patients, particularly when combined with chemotherapy.[101] Hart and colleagues[102] plotted posttreatment FDG uptake against radiation dose in the lung for subjects with esophageal cancer, and found a linear relationship. Using logistic regression analysis, they found that increases in both mean lung dose and the steepness of the uptake-dose curve were associated with an increased probability of radiation-induced pneumonitis. They found that there was much inter-subject variation in the steepness of the uptake-dose curve. That this parameter correlates with risk of pneumonitis risk may indicate that it is a good indicator of the relative radiation-sensitivity of individual patients. The same research group recently published similar results for subjects with lung cancer.[103] The use of 4D PET may have reduced some of the uncertainties in these results, although this was not studied.

RT can result in treatment-associated heart disease for patients treated for a range of cancers, including lymphoma, breast cancer, and lung cancer.[104,105] Patients treated for Hodgkin lymphoma are particularly at risk, and cardiovascular death is the main noncancer cause among long-term survivors of these treatments.[106] In fact, subclinical cardiac abnormalities are found in up to 50% of patients,[104] although clinical abnormalities (congestive heart failure, arrhythmia, autonomic dysfunction) are much less common. Single-photon emission computed tomography (SPECT) has been used to quantify radiation-induced cardiac changes and there is interest in the use of PET to quantify regional myocardial perfusion and the impact of RT.[105] In 2007, Zophel and colleagues[107] presented a case-report showing that FGD PET uptake increased in the parts of the myocardium that received in excess of 35 Gy during chemoradiotherapy for esophageal cancer 4 years earlier. More recently, Konski and colleagues[108] retrospectively reviewed data from 102 patients treated using chemoradiotherapy for esophageal cancer and found no correlation between changes in myocardial SUV and cardiac toxicity for this initial study.

SUMMARY

RT is at a point at which accurate delineation of the tumor is critical and identification of subvolumes that may be treatment-resistant can be accurately planned and treated. The introduction of 4D PET-CT facilitates this for tumors affected by respiratory motion. Thus, although this is still a research topic, the tools and techniques are in place for their practical clinical implementation over the next few years. Also, there is increasing evidence that PET can play an important part in predicting and assessing dose response, both for tumors and normal tissues. The introduction of 4D PET can potentially improve the quality of these data.

ACKNOWLEDGMENTS

The authors would like to thank Dr Michalis Aristophanous for discussions during the writing of this article.

REFERENCES

1. International Commission on Radiation Units, Measurements. Prescribing, recording, and reporting photon beam therapy. Bethesda (MD): International Commission on Radiation Units and Measurements; 1993.
2. International Commission on Radiation Units, Measurements. Prescribing, recording, and reporting photon beam therapy. Bethesda (MD): International Commission on Radiation Units and Measurements; 1999.
3. Mutaf YD, Brinkmann DH. Optimization of internal margin to account for dosimetric effects of respiratory motion. Int J Radiat Oncol Biol Phys 2008; 70(5):1561–70.
4. van Herk M. Errors and margins in radiotherapy. Semin Radiat Oncol 2004;14(1):52–64.
5. Winey B, Wagar M, Ebe K, et al. Effect of respiratory trace shape on optimal treatment margin. Med Phys 2011;38(6):3125–9.
6. Seppenwoolde Y, Shirato H, Kitamura K, et al. Precise and real-time measurement of 3D tumor motion in lung due to breathing and heartbeat, measured during radiotherapy. Int J Radiat Oncol Biol Phys 2002;53(4):822–34.
7. Langen KM, Jones DT. Organ motion and its management. Int J Radiat Oncol Biol Phys 2001; 50(1):265–78.
8. Ezzell GA, Galvin JM, Low D, et al. Guidance document on delivery, treatment planning, and clinical implementation of IMRT: report of the IMRT Subcommittee of the AAPM Radiation Therapy Committee. Med Phys 2003;30(8):2089–115.
9. Ten Haken RK, Lawrence TS. The clinical application of intensity-modulated radiation therapy. Semin Radiat Oncol 2006;16(4):224–31.
10. Otto K. Volumetric modulated arc therapy: IMRT in a single gantry arc. Med Phys 2008;35(1):310–7.
11. Verbakel WF, Senan S, Cuijpers JP, et al. Rapid delivery of stereotactic radiotherapy for peripheral lung tumors using volumetric intensity-modulated arcs. Radiother Oncol 2009;93(1):122–4.
12. Bissonnette JP, Balter PA, Dong L, et al. Quality assurance for image-guided radiation therapy utilizing CT-based technologies: a report of the AAPM TG-179. Med Phys 2012;39(4):1946–63.
13. van Herk M. Different styles of image-guided radiotherapy. Semin Radiat Oncol 2007;17(4):258–67.
14. Kitamura K, Court LE, Dong L. Comparison of imaging modalities for image-guided radiation therapy (IGRT). Nihon Igaku Hoshasen Gakkai Zasshi 2003;63(9):574–8 [in Japanese].
15. Underberg RW, Lagerwaard FJ, Slotman BJ, et al. Benefit of respiration-gated stereotactic radiotherapy for stage I lung cancer: an analysis of 4DCT datasets. Int J Radiat Oncol Biol Phys 2005;62(2):554–60.
16. Keall PJ, Mageras GS, Balter JM, et al. The management of respiratory motion in radiation oncology report of AAPM Task Group 76. Med Phys 2006;33(10):3874–900.
17. Moorrees J, Bezak E. Four dimensional CT imaging: a review of current technologies and modalities. Australas Phys Eng Sci Med 2012; 35(1):9–23.
18. Rietzel E, Liu AK, Doppke KP, et al. Design of 4D treatment planning target volumes. Int J Radiat Oncol Biol Phys 2006;66(1):287–95.
19. Rietzel E, Pan T, Chen GT. Four-dimensional computed tomography: image formation and clinical protocol. Med Phys 2005;32(4):874–89.
20. Guckenberger M, Richter A, Boda-Heggemann J, et al. Motion compensation in radiotherapy. Crit Rev Biomed Eng 2012;40(3):187–97.
21. Nelson C, Starkschall G, Balter P, et al. Assessment of lung tumor motion and setup uncertainties using implanted fiducials. Int J Radiat Oncol Biol Phys 2007;67(3):915–23.
22. Bortfeld T, Jiang SB, Rietzel E. Effects of motion on the total dose distribution. Semin Radiat Oncol 2004;14(1):41–51.
23. Chang JY, Cox JD. Improving radiation conformality in the treatment of non-small cell lung cancer. Semin Radiat Oncol 2010;20(3):171–7.
24. MacManus M, Nestle U, Rosenzweig KE, et al. Use of PET and PET/CT for radiation therapy planning: IAEA expert report 2006–2007. Radiother Oncol 2009;91(1):85–94.
25. Nestle U, Weber W, Hentschel M, et al. Biological imaging in radiation therapy: role of positron emission tomography. Phys Med Biol 2009;54(1):R1–25.
26. Ford EC, Herman J, Yorke E, et al. 18F-FDG PET/CT for image-guided and intensity-modulated radiotherapy. J Nucl Med 2009;50(10):1655–65.
27. Muijs CT, Schreurs LM, Busz DM, et al. Consequences of additional use of PET information for target volume delineation and radiotherapy dose

distribution for esophageal cancer. Radiother Oncol 2009;93(3):447–53.

28. Wang H, Vees H, Miralbell R, et al. 18F-fluorocholine PET-guided target volume delineation techniques for partial prostate re-irradiation in local recurrent prostate cancer. Radiother Oncol 2009; 93(2):220–5.

29. Bradley J, Thorstad WL, Mutic S, et al. Impact of FDG-PET on radiation therapy volume delineation in non-small-cell lung cancer. Int J Radiat Oncol Biol Phys 2004;59(1):78–86.

30. Moule RN, Kayani I, Moinuddin SA, et al. The potential advantages of (18)FDG PET/CT-based target volume delineation in radiotherapy planning of head and neck cancer. Radiother Oncol 2010; 97(2):189–93.

31. Nestle U, Kremp S, Schaefer-Schuler A, et al. Comparison of different methods for delineation of 18F-FDG PET-positive tissue for target volume definition in radiotherapy of patients with non-Small cell lung cancer. J Nucl Med 2005;46(8): 1342–8.

32. Milker-Zabel S, Zabel-du Bois A, Henze M, et al. Improved target volume definition for fractionated stereotactic radiotherapy in patients with intracranial meningiomas by correlation of CT, MRI, and [68Ga]-DOTATOC-PET. Int J Radiat Oncol Biol Phys 2006;65(1):222–7.

33. Astner ST, Bundschuh RA, Beer AJ, et al. Assessment of tumor volumes in skull base glomus tumors using Gluc-Lys[(18)F]-TOCA positron emission tomography. Int J Radiat Oncol Biol Phys 2009; 73(4):1135–40.

34. Vanderstraeten B, Duthoy W, De Gersem W, et al. [18F]fluoro-deoxy-glucose positron emission tomography ([18F]FDG-PET) voxel intensity-based intensity-modulated radiation therapy (IMRT) for head and neck cancer. Radiother Oncol 2006; 79(3):249–58.

35. Grosu AL, Piert M, Weber WA, et al. Positron emission tomography for radiation treatment planning. Strahlenther Onkol 2005;181(8):483–99.

36. Nestle U, Walter K, Schmidt S, et al. 18F-deoxyglucose positron emission tomography (FDG-PET) for the planning of radiotherapy in lung cancer: high impact in patients with atelectasis. Int J Radiat Oncol Biol Phys 1999;44(3):593–7.

37. Deniaud-Alexandre E, Touboul E, Lerouge D, et al. Impact of computed tomography and 18F-deoxyglucose coincidence detection emission tomography image fusion for optimization of conformal radiotherapy in non-small-cell lung cancer. Int J Radiat Oncol Biol Phys 2005;63(5): 1432–41.

38. Caldwell CB, Mah K, Skinner M, et al. Can PET provide the 3D extent of tumor motion for individualized internal target volumes? A phantom study of the limitations of CT and the promise of PET. Int J Radiat Oncol Biol Phys 2003;55(5):1381–93.

39. Caldwell CB, Mah K, Ung YC, et al. Observer variation in contouring gross tumor volume in patients with poorly defined non-small-cell lung tumors on CT: the impact of 18FDG-hybrid PET fusion. Int J Radiat Oncol Biol Phys 2001;51(4):923–31.

40. Fox JL, Rengan R, O'Meara W, et al. Does registration of PET and planning CT images decrease interobserver and intraobserver variation in delineating tumor volumes for non-small-cell lung cancer? Int J Radiat Oncol Biol Phys 2005;62(1):70–5.

41. Mac Manus MP, Hicks RJ, Ball DL, et al. F-18 fluorodeoxyglucose positron emission tomography staging in radical radiotherapy candidates with nonsmall cell lung carcinoma: powerful correlation with survival and high impact on treatment. Cancer 2001;92(4):886–95.

42. De Ruysscher D, Nestle U, Jeraj R, et al. PET scans in radiotherapy planning of lung cancer. Lung Cancer 2012;75(2):141–5.

43. Bradley JD, Bae K, Choi N, et al. A phase II comparative study of gross tumor volume definition with or without PET/CT fusion in dosimetric planning for non–small-cell lung cancer (NSCLC): primary analysis of radiation therapy oncology group (RTOG) 0515. Int J Radiat Oncol Biol Phys 2009;75(Suppl 3):S2.

44. Bradley J, Bae K, Choi N, et al. A phase II comparative study of gross tumor volume definition with or without PET/CT fusion in dosimetric planning for non-small-cell lung cancer (NSCLC): primary analysis of Radiation Therapy Oncology Group (RTOG) 0515. Int J Radiat Oncol Biol Phys 2012;82(1): 435–441.e1.

45. Schinagl DA, Hoffmann AL, Vogel WV, et al. Can FDG-PET assist in radiotherapy target volume definition of metastatic lymph nodes in head-and-neck cancer? Radiother Oncol 2009;91(1):95–100.

46. Paulino AC, Koshy M, Howell R, et al. Comparison of CT- and FDG-PET-defined gross tumor volume in intensity-modulated radiotherapy for head-and-neck cancer. Int J Radiat Oncol Biol Phys 2005; 61(5):1385–92.

47. Scarfone C, Lavely WC, Cmelak AJ, et al. Prospective feasibility trial of radiotherapy target definition for head and neck cancer using 3-dimensional PET and CT imaging. J Nucl Med 2004;45(4): 543–52.

48. Dietl B, Marienhagen J, Kuhnel T, et al. FDG-PET in radiotherapy treatment planning of advanced head and neck cancer—a prospective clinical analysis. Auris Nasus Larynx 2006;33(3):303–9.

49. Boellaard R, O'Doherty MJ, Weber WA, et al. FDG PET and PET/CT: EANM procedure guidelines for tumour PET imaging: version 1.0. Eur J Nucl Med Mol Imaging 2010;37(1):181–200.

50. Delbeke D, Coleman RE, Guiberteau MJ, et al. Procedure guideline for tumor imaging with 18F-FDG PET/CT 1.0. J Nucl Med 2006;47(5): 885–95.

51. Bettinardi V, Picchio M, Di Muzio N, et al. Detection and compensation of organ/lesion motion using 4D-PET/CT respiratory gated acquisition techniques. Radiother Oncol 2010;96(3):311–6.

52. Zaidi H, El Naqa I. PET-guided delineation of radiation therapy treatment volumes: a survey of image segmentation techniques. Eur J Nucl Med Mol Imaging 2010;37(11):2165–87.

53. Mac Manus MP, Hicks RJ. The role of positron emission tomography/computed tomography in radiation therapy planning for patients with lung cancer. Semin Nucl Med 2012;42(5):308–19.

54. IAEA. The role of PET/CT in treatment planning for cancer patient treatment. Vienna (Austria): IAEA; 2008.

55. Soret M, Bacharach SL, Buvat I. Partial-volume effect in PET tumor imaging. J Nucl Med 2007; 48(6):932–45.

56. Bayne M, Hicks RJ, Everitt S, et al. Reproducibility of "intelligent" contouring of gross tumor volume in non-small-cell lung cancer on PET/CT images using a standardized visual method. Int J Radiat Oncol Biol Phys 2010;77(4):1151–7.

57. Chen CH, Muzic RF Jr, Nelson AD, et al. Simultaneous recovery of size and radioactivity concentration of small spheroids with PET data. J Nucl Med 1999;40(1):118–30.

58. King AD. Multimodality imaging of head and neck cancer. Cancer Imaging 2007;7(Spec No A): S37–46.

59. Hof H, Rhein B, Haering P, et al. 4D-CT-based target volume definition in stereotactic radiotherapy of lung tumours: comparison with a conventional technique using individual margins. Radiother Oncol 2009;93(3):419–23.

60. Dawood M, Buther F, Stegger L, et al. Optimal number of respiratory gates in positron emission tomography: a cardiac patient study. Med Phys 2009;36(5):1775–84.

61. Bettinardi V, Rapisarda E, Gilardi MC. Number of partitions (gates) needed to obtain motion-free images in a respiratory gated 4D-PET/CT study as a function of the lesion size and motion displacement. Med Phys 2009;36(12): 5547–58.

62. van Elmpt W, Hamill J, Jones J, et al. Optimal gating compared to 3D and 4D PET reconstruction for characterization of lung tumours. Eur J Nucl Med Mol Imaging 2011;38(5):843–55.

63. Bettinardi V, Picchio M, Di Muzio N, et al. Motion management in positron emission tomography/computed tomography for radiation treatment planning. Semin Nucl Med 2012;42(5):289–307.

64. Nehmeh SA, Erdi YE. Respiratory motion in positron emission tomography/computed tomography: a review. Semin Nucl Med 2008;38(3): 167–76.

65. Schafers KP, Stegger L. Combined imaging of molecular function and morphology with PET/CT and SPECT/CT: image fusion and motion correction. Basic Res Cardiol 2008;103(2):191–9.

66. Li T, Thorndyke B, Schreibmann E, et al. Model-based image reconstruction for four-dimensional PET. Med Phys 2006;33(5):1288–98.

67. Qiao F, Pan T, Clark JW Jr, et al. A motion-incorporated reconstruction method for gated PET studies. Phys Med Biol 2006;51(15):3769–83.

68. Chang G, Chang T, Pan T, et al. Implementation of an automated respiratory amplitude gating technique for PET/CT: clinical evaluation. J Nucl Med 2010;51(1):16–24.

69. Grosu AL, Souvatzoglou M, Roper B, et al. Hypoxia imaging with FAZA-PET and theoretical considerations with regard to dose painting for individualization of radiotherapy in patients with head and neck cancer. Int J Radiat Oncol Biol Phys 2007; 69(2):541–51.

70. Seppala J, Seppanen M, Arponen E, et al. Carbon-11 acetate PET/CT based dose escalated IMRT in prostate cancer. Radiother Oncol 2009;93(2): 234–40.

71. Pinkawa M, Attieh C, Piroth MD, et al. Dose-escalation using intensity-modulated radiotherapy for prostate cancer–evaluation of the dose distribution with and without 18F-choline PET-CT detected simultaneous integrated boost. Radiother Oncol 2009;93(2):213–9.

72. Lin Z, Mechalakos J, Nehmeh S, et al. The influence of changes in tumor hypoxia on dose-painting treatment plans based on 18F-FMISO positron emission tomography. Int J Radiat Oncol Biol Phys 2008;70(4):1219–28.

73. Madani I, Duthoy W, Derie C, et al. Positron emission tomography-guided, focal-dose escalation using intensity-modulated radiotherapy for head and neck cancer. Int J Radiat Oncol Biol Phys 2007;68(1):126–35.

74. Sovik A, Malinen E, Skogmo HK, et al. Radiotherapy adapted to spatial and temporal variability in tumor hypoxia. Int J Radiat Oncol Biol Phys 2007;68(5):1496–504.

75. Thorwarth D, Eschmann SM, Paulsen F, et al. Hypoxia dose painting by numbers: a planning study. Int J Radiat Oncol Biol Phys 2007;68(1): 291–300.

76. Chao KS, Bosch WR, Mutic S, et al. A novel approach to overcome hypoxic tumor resistance: Cu-ATSM-guided intensity-modulated radiation therapy. Int J Radiat Oncol Biol Phys 2001;49(4): 1171–82.

77. Sovik A, Malinen E, Olsen DR. Strategies for biologic image-guided dose escalation: a review. Int J Radiat Oncol Biol Phys 2009;73(3):650–8.

78. Alber M, Paulsen F, Eschmann SM, et al. On biologically conformal boost dose optimization. Phys Med Biol 2003;48(2):N31–5.

79. Bentzen SM. Theragnostic imaging for radiation oncology: dose-painting by numbers. Lancet Oncol 2005;6(2):112–7.

80. Petit SF, Aerts HJ, van Loon JG, et al. Metabolic control probability in tumour subvolumes or how to guide tumour dose redistribution in non-small cell lung cancer (NSCLC): an exploratory clinical study. Radiother Oncol 2009;91(3):393–8.

81. Bowen SR, Flynn RT, Bentzen SM, et al. On the sensitivity of IMRT dose optimization to the mathematical form of a biological imaging-based prescription function. Phys Med Biol 2009;54(6):1483–501.

82. Aristophanous M, Yap JT, Killoran JH, et al. Four-dimensional positron emission tomography: implications for dose painting of high-uptake regions. Int J Radiat Oncol Biol Phys 2011;80(3):900–8.

83. Yang Y, Wu Y, Qi J, et al. A prototype PET scanner with DOI-encoding detectors. J Nucl Med 2008;49(7):1132–40.

84. Reader AJ. The promise of new PET image reconstruction. Phys Med 2008;24(2):49–56.

85. Karp JS, Surti S, Daube-Witherspoon ME, et al. Benefit of time-of-flight in PET: experimental and clinical results. J Nucl Med 2008;49(3):462–70.

86. Clarke K, Taremi M, Dahele M, et al. Stereotactic body radiotherapy (SBRT) for non-small cell lung cancer (NSCLC): is FDG-PET a predictor of outcome? Radiother Oncol 2012;104(1):62–6.

87. Takeda A, Yokosuka N, Ohashi T, et al. The maximum standardized uptake value (SUVmax) on FDG-PET is a strong predictor of local recurrence for localized non-small-cell lung cancer after stereotactic body radiotherapy (SBRT). Radiother Oncol 2011;101(2):291–7.

88. Aerts HJ, van Baardwijk AA, Petit SF, et al. Identification of residual metabolic-active areas within individual NSCLC tumours using a pre-radiotherapy 18Fluorodeoxyglucose-PET-CT scan. Radiother Oncol 2009;91(3):386–92.

89. Petit SF, van Elmpt WJ, Oberije CJ, et al. [18F]fluorodeoxyglucose uptake patterns in lung before radiotherapy identify areas more susceptible to radiation-induced lung toxicity in non-small-cell lung cancer patients. Int J Radiat Oncol Biol Phys 2011;81(3):698–705.

90. De Ruysscher D, Houben A, Aerts HJ, et al. Increased (18)F-deoxyglucose uptake in the lung during the first weeks of radiotherapy is correlated with subsequent Radiation-Induced Lung Toxicity (RILT): a prospective pilot study. Radiother Oncol 2009;91(3):415–20.

91. McCloskey P, Ford V, Bissonnette J, et al. PO-0745 can FDG pet during the course of radiation therapy for lung cancer predict for esophagitis and pneumonitis outcome? Radiother Oncol 2012;103(Suppl 1(0)):S289.

92. Werner-Wasik M, Yorke E, Deasy J, et al. Radiation dose-volume effects in the esophagus. Int J Radiat Oncol Biol Phys 2010;76(Suppl 3):S86–93.

93. Dieleman EM, Senan S, Vincent A, et al. Four-dimensional computed tomographic analysis of esophageal mobility during normal respiration. Int J Radiat Oncol Biol Phys 2007;67(3):775–80.

94. Werner-Wasik M, Xiao Y, Pequignot E, et al. Assessment of lung cancer response after nonoperative therapy: tumor diameter, bidimensional product, and volume. A serial CT scan-based study. Int J Radiat Oncol Biol Phys 2001;51(1):56–61.

95. Mac Manus M, Hicks RJ. The Use of Positron Emission Tomography (PET) in the staging/evaluation, treatment, and follow-up of patients with lung cancer: a critical review. Int J Radiat Oncol Biol Phys 2008;72(5):1298–306.

96. Mac Manus MP, Hicks RJ, Matthews JP, et al. Positron emission tomography is superior to computed tomography scanning for response-assessment after radical radiotherapy or chemoradiotherapy in patients with non–small-cell lung cancer. J Clin Oncol 2003;21(7):1285–92.

97. Bury T, Corhay JL, Duysinx B, et al. Value of FDG-PET in detecting residual or recurrent non-small cell lung cancer. Eur Respir J 1999;14(6):1376–80.

98. Aristophanous M, Yong Y, Yap JT, et al. Evaluating FDG uptake changes between pre and post therapy respiratory gated PET scans. Radiother Oncol 2012;102(3):377–82.

99. Wahl RL, Jacene H, Kasamon Y, et al. From RECIST to PERCIST: evolving considerations for PET response criteria in solid tumors. J Nucl Med 2009;50(Suppl 1):122S–50S.

100. Young H, Baum R, Cremerius U, et al. Measurement of clinical and subclinical tumour response using [18F]-fluorodeoxyglucose and positron emission tomography: review and 1999 EORTC recommendations. European Organization for Research and Treatment of Cancer (EORTC) PET Study Group. Eur J Cancer 1999;35(13):1773–82.

101. Marks LB, Bentzen SM, Deasy JO, et al. Radiation dose-volume effects in the lung. Int J Radiat Oncol Biol Phys 2010;76(Suppl 3):S70–6.

102. Hart JP, McCurdy MR, Ezhil M, et al. Radiation pneumonitis: correlation of toxicity with pulmonary metabolic radiation response. Int J Radiat Oncol Biol Phys 2008;71(4):967–71.

103. McCurdy MR, Castillo R, Martinez J, et al. [18F]-FDG uptake dose-response correlates with radiation pneumonitis in lung cancer patients. Radiother Oncol 2012;104(1):52–7.

104. Gagliardi G, Constine LS, Moiseenko V, et al. Radiation dose-volume effects in the heart. Int J Radiat Oncol Biol Phys 2010;76(Suppl 3):S77–85.

105. Robbins ME, Brunso-Bechtold JK, Peiffer AM, et al. Imaging radiation-induced normal tissue injury. Radiat Res 2012;177(4):449–66.

106. Favier O, Heutte N, Stamatoullas-Bastard A, et al. Survival after Hodgkin lymphoma: causes of death and excess mortality in patients treated in 8 consecutive trials. Cancer 2009;115(8):1680–91.

107. Zophel K, Holzel C, Dawel M, et al. PET/CT demonstrates increased myocardial FDG uptake following irradiation therapy. Eur J Nucl Med Mol Imaging 2007;34(8):1322–3.

108. Konski A, Li T, Christensen M, et al. Symptomatic cardiac toxicity is predicted by dosimetric and patient factors rather than changes in 18F-FDG PET determination of myocardial activity after chemoradiotherapy for esophageal cancer. Radiother Oncol 2012;104(1):72–7.

Modeling and Simulation of 4D PET-CT and PET-MR Images

Charalampos Tsoumpas, MPhys, MSc, DIC, PhD[a],*,
Anastasios Gaitanis, MSc, PhD[b]

KEYWORDS

- Digital phantoms • Simulation software • Kinetic modeling • Physiologic modeling
- Respiratory and cardiac motion • Medical imaging • Positron emission tomography

KEY POINTS

- Digital phantoms used for simulation in hybrid PET imaging are usually developed from segmented CT scans or MR images.
- MR or CT dynamic images can be used for realistic three-dimensional motion simulation of human body motion in PET imaging.
- Data simulation and PET modeling software tools are necessary for the simulation of physical processes and data acquisition, which are based on either Monte Carlo or analytical methods.
- Future computational four-dimensional PET-CT/MR imaging simulations may include multiscale and multiphysics mathematical modeling derived from physiologic measurements of organs.
- Statistical iterative reconstruction techniques include physics models, statistics, and potentially tracer kinetics of the PET acquisition to make the inverse problem more consistent.

INTRODUCTION

The growing success of radiologic imaging has led to the evolution of new molecular imaging modalities that assist in improving diagnosis and staging of diseases. A successful commercial molecular imaging device is the PET scanner combined with computerized tomography (CT)[1] or more recently with MR imaging scanners.[2–4] The new PET-CT/MR imaging systems are among the most elegant devices available in the clinic. This article provides a critical discussion on the current advances achieved in modeling and simulation of four-dimensional PET-CT/MR images from the PET perspective. In addition, it provides a vision on how recent advances in biomechanics, biophysics, and biochemistry may help improve the realism and accuracy towards personalized four-dimensional PET modeling and simulation.

The improvement in PET image quality depends on the development of scanners with better

Funding: Dr C. Tsoumpas' work was mainly funded by the European Union under two 7th framework programs: HYPERImage (No: 201,651, http://www.hybrid-pet-mr.eu) and SUBLIMA (No: 241,711, http://www.sublima-pet-mr.eu). Dr A. Gaitanis was supported in part from the COST action TD1007 (http://www.pet-mri.eu) entitled "Bimodal PET-MRI molecular imaging technologies and applications for in vivo monitoring of disease and biologic processes." Dr C. Tsoumpas acknowledges additional financial support from the Department of Health via the National Institute for Health Research (NIHR) comprehensive Biomedical Research Center award to Guy's & St Thomas' NHS Foundation Trust in partnership with King's College London and King's College Hospital NHS Foundation Trust.

[a] Division of Imaging Sciences and Biomedical Engineering, Department of Biomedical Engineering, King's College London, King's Health Partners, St. Thomas' Hospital, London SE1 7EH, UK; [b] Department of Biomedical Technology, Biomedical Research Foundation of the Academy of Athens, Soranou Efessiou 4, Athens 11527, Greece
* Corresponding author.
E-mail address: charalampos.tsoumpas@kcl.ac.uk

PET Clin 8 (2013) 95–110
http://dx.doi.org/10.1016/j.cpet.2012.10.003
1556-8598/13/$ – see front matter Crown Copyright © 2013 Published by Elsevier Inc. All rights reserved.

hardware and software capabilities. Several factors may cause degradation of image quality and accuracy. For example, the subject's motion and the potentially fast tracer kinetics may generate images with poor quantification information. The estimation of their effects can be examined using realistic four-dimensional simulations. Furthermore, accurate and realistic simulations of the four-dimensional PET acquisition can help beyond the validation and evaluation performance of hardware and software. PET statistical iterative reconstruction approximates the measurement with modeling of physics (eg, scatter, detector response[5]), patient motion[6] and anatomy,[7] statistics,[8] and potentially tracer kinetics,[9] which helps to make the inverse problem less ill-posed and obtain more consistent results. An improved acquisition model will increase the accuracy and precision of the estimated physiologic parameters of interest. Therefore, computational simulations offer a pathway to the characterization of the acquisition process from the injection of the tracer to the detection of the photons to derive physiologic information.

During the early days of emission tomography research, four-dimensional simulations were not practical because of the highly demanding computational power requirements. However, with the development of modern computers possessing large processing capabilities four-dimensional simulations have become feasible. For the successful generation of these simulations, realistic information is necessary. The first aspect is the four-dimensional computational phantom, which usually consists of a (realistic) three-dimensional numerical phantom; realistic three-dimensional motion fields; and pharmacokinetic/physiologic properties for different tissues. The second aspect is the data simulation software that includes the scanner geometry and physical characteristics. This article discusses these aspects in detail.

FOUR-DIMENSIONAL COMPUTATIONAL PHANTOMS
Realistic Three-Dimensional Numerical Phantoms

Numerical phantoms have been used since the 1960s and have evolved alongside the revolution of computed medical imaging.[10] Undoubtedly, the computational phantoms have been very useful in emission tomography.[11] They offer the convenience of virtually evaluating different scenarios of human anatomy and physiology, enabling the most optimal design of acquisition protocols, image reconstruction, and processing

methods[12] to be developed. An example of this kind of phantom is the VIP-Man model, which includes several organs.[13] The standard approach to designing a realistic computational phantom is the segmentation and combination of multiple high-resolution MR or CT images.[14–17] For example, Zubal and coworkers[18] designed the Voxelman, one of the most widely used numerical phantoms in emission tomography. However, voxelized phantoms have some limitations, especially in cases where walled organs have been segmented or body tissues have been altered. Mesh phantoms have been recommended as the next generation of advanced computational phantoms that can avoid these limitations.

An example of the most widely used mathematical phantom is the cardiac torso MCAT[19] and its evolution the XCAT[20] (also known as NCAT) and PCAT.[21] The MCAT is based on geometric primitives. XCAT allows much more realistic modeling of cardiac anatomy than MCAT and expands its applications beyond nuclear medicine.[22] PCAT is a four-dimensional perfusion cardiac-torso phantom[21] designed for dynamic perfusion nuclear medicine simulation studies. This family of phantoms belongs to a new generation, the so-called hybrid phantoms, where the organs are described using volumetric measurements and mathematical models. For example, in the case of the most recent version of this phantom, the XCAT, the human body is based on a very high-resolution anatomic datasets, the Visible Male and Female from the National Library of Medicine (http://www.nlm.nih.gov/research/visible/visible_human.html) as shown in **Fig. 1**. The mathematical model that describes the phantom is the nonuniform rational B-splines. These are mathematical models used in computer graphics for the generation and representation of curves and surfaces. Their advantage is that they offer great flexibility and precision for handling analytic and freeform shapes and they have been used by several research groups for the development of hybrid patient-dependent phantoms (**Fig. 2**).[23] In particular, the XCAT phantom represents more than 9000 regions of the human body in detail. In addition, one version has been expanded such that it includes the anatomies of 30 organs of the grown child until the age of 16 months.[24] The flexibility in fitting the XCAT phantom to existing patient anatomic data offers new opportunities for exploiting four-dimensional simulations with realistic anatomic variability. The high-resolution detail of the phantom allows for the simulation of CT acquisitions,[22] as shown in **Fig. 3**. Furthermore, **Fig. 4** illustrates an example of a dynamic PET cardiac image based on the

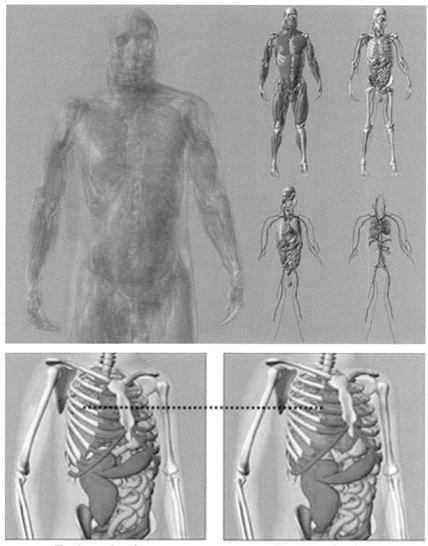

End-expiration   **End-inspiration**

Fig. 1. Human anatomy of the extended NCAT or XCAT phantoms. Such details as circulatory system, organs, glands, skeleton, muscles, and respiratory motion are illustrated (*top*). Respiratory positions at end-expiration and end-inspiration of the enhanced four-dimensional XCAT are illustrated (*bottom left and bottom right*, respectively). (*From* Segars WP, Tsui BM. MCAT to XCAT: the evolution of 4-D computerized phantoms for imaging research. Proc IEEE 2009;97(12):1960–3, http://dx.doi.org/10.1109/JPROC.2009.2022417; with permission.)

PCAT phantom. Finally, Segars and his colleagues[25] extended their methodology to support the development of small animal imaging research and developed the dynamic rodent phantom called MOBY, which includes respiratory and cardiac motion based on a mouse.

Another type of hybrid computational phantom is illustrated in **Fig. 5.**[26] These phantoms model overweight and underweight individuals and they can be used to optimize four-dimensional PET acquisition protocols by simulating with higher complexity multiple patients or longitudinal PET imaging sessions that may be subject to functional and anatomic variability. Similarly, another series of hybrid-voxel phantoms with variable age (eg, newborn, 1, 5, 10, and 15 year old, and adult male and female) has been developed by Bolch at the University of Florida and Lee at the National Cancer Institute.[27] Currently, these phantoms do not necessarily include respiratory or cardiac motion, but this could potentially be adapted in the future.

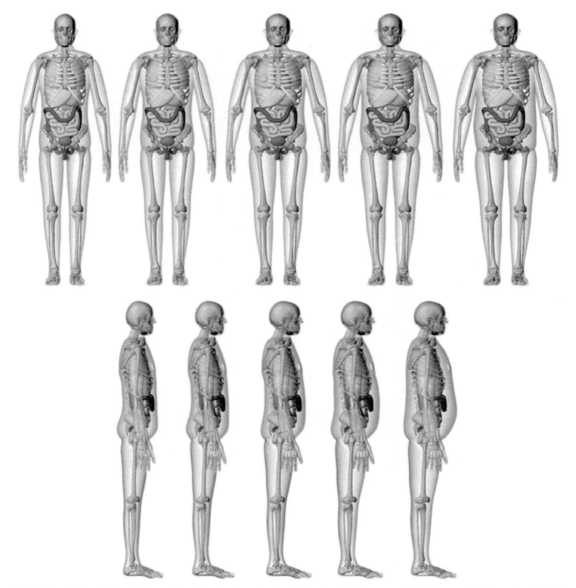

Fig. 2. Frontal and lateral views of patient-dependent adult male phantoms as at 50th percentile standing height and 10th, 25th, 50th, 75th, and 90th percentile body mass. (*From* Johnson PB, Whalen SR, Wayson M, et al. Hybrid patient-dependent phantoms covering statistical distributions of body morphometry in the U.S. adult and pediatric population. Proc IEEE 2009;97(12):2068, http://dx.doi.org/10.1109/JPROC.2009.2032855; with permission.)

One of the main disadvantages of most three-dimensional numerical phantoms is that they do not include a realistic representation of the patient's variable function and anatomy caused by disease. Usually, these phantoms are designed from healthy volunteers or from single patients. The development of representative anatomic and functional disease models is an open research area in modeling and simulation of whole-body PET images.

Realistic Motion

Realistic simulation of the human body motion that occurs during acquisition is highly complicated. The motion of each point of the human body can be approximated by a normal periodic pattern with potential variation in respiration[28] and cardiac cycle, combined with body repositioning (ie, bulk movement). Additional types of motion exist, such as peristalsis,[29] prostate, and bladder motion,[30]

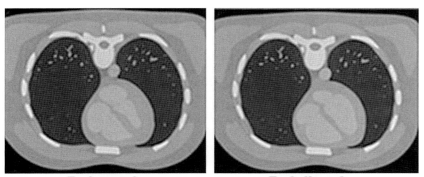

End-systole   **End-diastole**

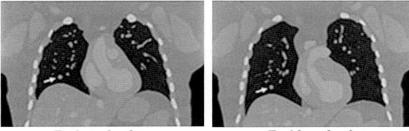

End-expiration   **End-inspiration**

Fig. 3. Cardiac-gated (*top*) and respiratory-gated (*bottom*) CT images generated using four-dimensional XCAT. (*From* Segars WP, Mahesh M, Beck TJ, et al. Realistic CT simulation using the four-dimensional XCAT phantom. Med Phys 2008;35(8):3806, http://dx.doi.org/10.1118/1.2955743; with permission.)

but these considerations are beyond the scope of this article. Any kind of motion that is of the same order as PET resolution can affect accuracy and potentially create a fundamental problem in count-limited acquisitions. The number of counts that correspond to the same position strongly depends on the changes of periodic motion magnitude, frequency, and other types of movement. To satisfactorily eliminate the motion artifacts, measurement of motion at least as accurate as the actual imaging system resolution is necessary.

Many researchers extract respiratory motion with sufficient temporal and spatial resolution from MR imaging[31] or CT acquisitions and use them for simulations of four-dimensional single-photon emission computed tomography (SPECT) and PET (**Fig. 6**).[32] These acquisitions are often combined with mathematical tools (eg, image registration)[33–35] to estimate the voxel displacements caused by motion of the subject. For example, Pollari and colleagues[16] used a method to simulate PET respiratory motion of thorax by measuring it with nonrigid registrations between different positions of the respiratory cycle. In the case of the state-of-the-art XCAT phantom (**Fig. 7**), dynamic information was obtained from multidetector CT scanners for the motion of the heart and several sets of respiratory-gated CT

images for the approximation of the respiratory cycle.[20] This phantom includes more than 100 time frames over the cardiac cycle and 20 time frames over the respiratory cycle. Compared with the previous version of the phantom, this has been a substantial improvement for simulation of respiratory motion because it has higher resolution and can include variable respiration signal modifiable to match real breathing pattern that can also be irregular. This is particularly complicated when imaging with PET because a few patients' respiratory traces have relatively small quiescent period fractions, which can yield results with large motion artifacts.[36]

Another problem especially in cardiac studies is the diaphragm motion: it can generate severe attenuation correction artifacts. As suggested by McQuaid and colleagues,[37] modeling motion of the diaphragm could help gate the CT images, which reduces the errors in the reconstructed PET images. A similar approach was followed in [^{13}N]-NH$_3$ PET-CT studies by Schleyer and colleagues,[38] who modeled the motion in CT using motion information from gated PET. Finally, little work has been performed for motion correction of preclinical PET imaging partly because the motion of rodents is not particularly large and it can be easily gated because of low variability.[39]

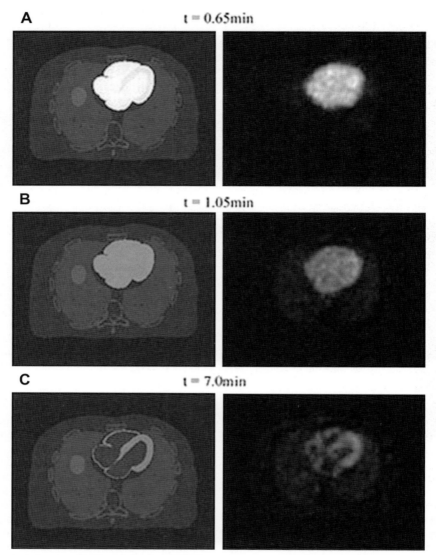

Fig. 4. Generated phantom (*left*) and simulated PET image sequence of a dynamic PCAT simulation with [82]Rb PET tracer. (*From* Fung G, Higuchi T, Park M, et al. Development of a four-dimensional digital phantom for tracer kinetic modeling and analysis of dynamic perfusion PET and SPECT simulation studies. In: 2011 IEEE Nuclear Science Symposium and Medical Imaging Conference. 2011. p. 4195, http://dx.doi.org/10.1109/NSSMIC.2011.6153803; with permission.)

Pharmacokinetic and Physiologic Modeling of Different Tissues

In addition to the standard respiratory and cardiac gated simulations, integration of pharmacokinetics is the next step that will increase the realism of PET simulations.[40] This is particularly interesting for development of new tracers. However, the level of complexity in modeling the biochemical aspects of a PET acquisition is much higher than physical and anatomic modeling. In practice, the radiotracer molecules follow the biochemical laws within the

entire physiologic system being imaged. Therefore, the tracer and the tissue properties of the entire body might need to be included in the model. Simulation of the biochemical interactions[41,42] could be theoretically described by quantum chemistry and require detailed understanding of the radiotracer chemical properties and their binding/interaction sites. A common molecular modeling software used in chemistry and drug development for this purpose is Gaussian v0.9 (http://www.gaussian.com/). This is designed to "advance molecular-level

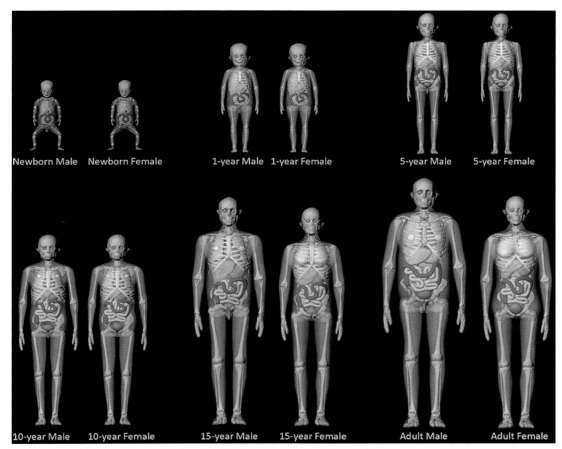

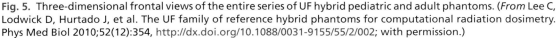

Fig. 5. Three-dimensional frontal views of the entire series of UF hybrid pediatric and adult phantoms. (*From* Lee C, Lodwick D, Hurtado J, et al. The UF family of reference hybrid phantoms for computational radiation dosimetry. Phys Med Biol 2010;52(12):354, http://dx.doi.org/10.1088/0031-9155/55/2/002; with permission.)

chemical research and help to study and predict the properties of molecules and reactions under a wide range of conditions."

Recently, an analytic biomathematical modeling approach to predict the in vivo performance of radioligands in the biologic system based on prior information from in vitro and in silico measurements has been suggested.[43,44] Nevertheless, the parent radiotracer is chemically active and can generate inside the body daughter radiotracer molecules, known also as the metabolites. Apart from augmenting the PET signal, these can also act as competitors of the parent tracer biochemical interactions. Therefore, in a few occasions the behavior of these molecules needs to be encapsulated within the pharmacokinetic simulation of a PET study.[45]

In addition to the traditional radiotracer investigations, there has been emerging interest in dual bimodal agents[46] where more complex biomolecules, such as proteins, peptides, and antibodies, can be labeled by a positron (or photon) emitter and imaged with PET (or SPECT) and CT–MR imaging. These multimodal agents have large size, and thus exhibit significantly slower kinetic behavior than standard PET tracers. Consequently, imaging requires long half-life radiotracers and potentially multiple acquisition sessions over hours or even days. Accurate longitudinal four-dimensional simulation of such studies would help to simplify the complicated imaging protocols needed for that type of investigation.

Finally, beyond dynamic PET simulations that include pharmacokinetic modeling, biomechanical tissue properties could be included in the next generation of dynamic phantoms as envisaged by Zaidi and Xu.[12] For example, the biomechanical properties of tumors,[47] blood flow, the main arteries (illustrated in **Fig. 8**),[48,49] and the cardiac cavities (**Figs. 9** and **10**).[50,51] The latter may become relevant in future hybrid four-dimensional PET simulations that could include multiscale and multiphysics mathematical modeling[52] derived from physiologic measurements of the heart, lungs,

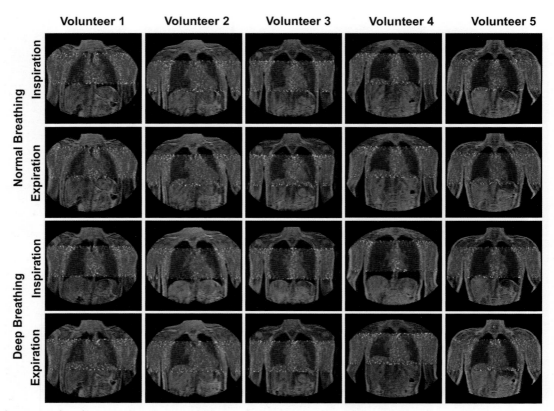

Fig. 6. Simulated PET-MR imaging acquisitions at inspiration and expiration phases of multiple volunteers with different respiration style. All images displayed in a fused style with the same color scale for PET and gray-scale for MR imaging. (*From* Tsoumpas C, Buerger C, King AP, et al. Fast generation of four-dimensional PET-MR data from real dynamic MR acquisitions. Phys Med Biol 2011;56(20):6610, http://dx.doi.org/10.1088/0031-9155/56/20/005; with permission.)

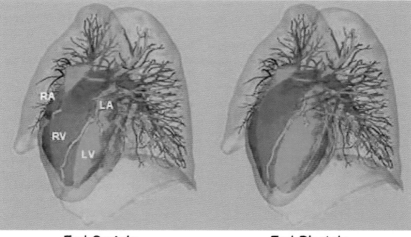

Fig. 7. Enhanced cardiac model of the four-dimensional XCAT based on multidetector CT. This model has been developed for males and females. LA, left atrium; LV, left ventricle; RA, right atrium; RV, right ventricle. (*From* Segars WP, Tsui BMW. MCAT to XCAT: the evolution of 4-D computerized phantoms for imaging research. Proc IEEE 2009;97(12):1962, http://dx.doi.org/10.1109/JPROC.2009.2022417; with permission.)

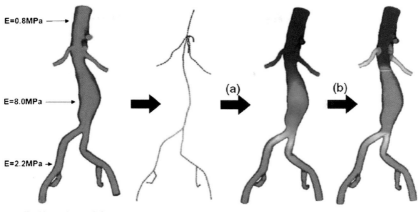

Fig. 8. Centerline-based (*a*) and surface-based (*b*) methods to assign variable wall properties. (*From* Xiong G, Figueroa C, Xiao N, et al. Simulation of blood flow in deformable vessels using subject-specific geometry and spatially varying wall properties. Int J Numer Method Biomed Eng 2010;27(7):1006, http://dx.doi.org/10.1002/cnm.1404; with permission.)

and other organs and specific disease-type tumors. Furthermore, as CT systems evolve, they may provide additional information in modeling blood flow properties and lung tissue function as recently demonstrated with a CT radiographic velocimetry technique (http://rsif.royalsociety publishing.org/content/9/74/2213/suppl/DC1).[53]

DATA SIMULATION SOFTWARE
Monte Carlo Simulators

The most common approach to simulate physical processes of PET or SPECT acquisition is based on Monte Carlo (MC) simulation. Several MC packages exist in medical imaging and they vary accordingly in precision, accuracy, and computational demand. Among these, GATE,[54] an open source software package (www.opengatecollaboration. org), is the most used. It can accommodate

different scanner geometries and has been validated for numerous PET and SPECT scanners.[55–57] Although GATE has the additional advantage of allowing modeling of time-dependent phenomena under realistic acquisition conditions, its main limitation is the extremely high computational demands for simulations without compromising statistical accuracy. Other packages that have supported PET research are SimSET[58] (http://depts. washington.edu/simset/html/user_guide/simset_asim_usergroup.html), PET-SORTEO[59] (Simulation of Realistic Tridimensional Emitting Objects; http://sorteo.cermep.fr/home.php), PeneloPET[60] (http://nuclear.fis.ucm.es/penelopet), Eidolon,[61] and GAMOS[62] (http://fismed.ciemat.es/GAMOS/). SimSET is based on MC simulations and aims to model the physical processes in emission tomography. It has a modular structure that allows one to speed up the simulation by reducing accuracy of the

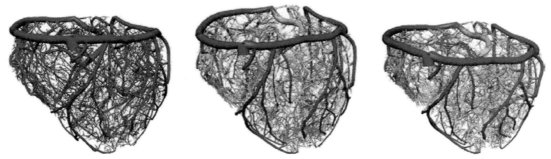

Fig. 9. Calculations of the normal stress for end-diastole, end-isovolumic contraction, and end-ejection scaled between 0 kPa (*dark blue*) and 10 kPa (*red*). (*From* Nordsletten DA, Niederer SA, Nash MP, et al. Coupling multiphysics models to cardiac mechanics. Prog Biophys Mol Biol 2011;104:85, http://dx.doi.org/10.1016/j.pbiomolbio. 2009.11.001; with permission.)

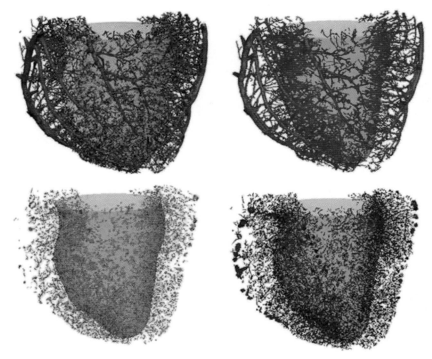

Fig. 10. The full vascular tree (*upper left*), vessels belonging to compartment one (*upper right*), vessels belonging to compartment two (*lower left*), and vessels belonging to compartment three (*lower right*). (*From* Cookson A, Lee J, Michler C, et al. A novel porous mechanical framework for modeling the interaction between coronary perfusion and myocardial mechanics. J Biomech 2012;104(1–3):853, http://dx.doi.org/10.1016/j.jbiomech.2011. 11.026; with permission.)

physical modeling. Moreover, the current version includes time-of-flight modeling and random coincidences. PET-SORTEO generates PET data from voxelized descriptions of tracer distributions taking into consideration the scanner's geometry, noise sources, and physical properties. Its output is normally in sinogram format but it has recently been extended into List-Mode.[63] Eidolon MC[64] has been designed to simulate fully three-dimensional cylindrical PET scanners on parallel computing. The software simulates the photon path length and the interaction processes within the phantoms and detectors. GAMOS is another recently developed simulation package, which like GATE is based on GEANT4 for medical imaging applications and has been designed with the aim to provide a flexible and well-validated toolkit.[65]

Generally, the MC packages can become faster at the expense of modeling accuracy and precision. Sometimes computational speed-up is achieved by the use of variance reduction techniques that may predict the correct physical response of the scanner, but without necessarily preserving the statistical properties of a real acquisition.[66] Additionally, even if several investigations have shown very good agreement with the acquired data, to the best of our knowledge none to date has investigated thoroughly their noise distribution and properties because of the extreme computational demand.

MC techniques are often used together with realistic numerical phantoms for several investigations. For example, they can be used to simulate numerous studies to develop a database (OncoPET_DB; https://www.creatis.insa-lyon.fr/oncoPET_DB) of clinical cases in whole-body PET.[67] An extension to this concept has been recently performed by Le Maitre and colleagues[68] who incorporated patient four-dimensional anatomic and functional variability of realistic whole-body FDG studies. The specific simulation was based on PET-SORTEO using the XCAT phantom, which was modified to fit actual CT scans of PET-CT patients. In addition, the phantom included inhomogeneous tumors and the effect of respiratory motion. In this way the simulations provide data with an extended spectrum of realism and they can be used as gold standard for future investigations. The objective of most of these simulations is the generation of realistic PET databases that would minimize computational cost.[67] An example of the simulated dataset was compared with the corresponding real PET-CT image, it is illustrated in **Fig. 11**. This offers the advantage to researchers to optimize their methodologies. However, the computational burden to repeat multiple realizations of a simulation can still be very high (ie, 70 hours for one realization of a static scan). A completely realistic and statistically accurate four-dimensional study for whole-body imaging that includes physiologic and anatomic variability is computationally demanding. Thus, there is still need for development of faster simulation toolkits.

Analytic Simulators

An attempt to address the need for computational speed is the development of fast analytic simulation packages. A rigorous approach has first been implemented by Ma and colleagues,[15,69] who has shown realistic simulations of brain PET data derived from MR imaging measurements. In these investigations analytic approaches to simulate different physical effects have been developed. In particular they demonstrated a simulation of real measurements including such effects as attenuation, scatter, random coincidences, detector variability and detector gaps, and statistical noise, showing that it is possible to satisfactorily simulate PET data with analytic techniques.

Another example of an analytic simulator is Analytic SIMulator[70] (ASIM; http://depts.washington. edu/asimuw/Info.html), an open-source software specifically designed for PET. ASIM provides several options, such as the simulation of emission data in two-dimensional or three-dimensional mode, attenuation correction, random and scatter events, detector blurring, normalization, and noise propagation. It has been used in various studies (eg, lesion detectability in response to various parameters).[71] An example of PET image simulation based on ASIM is illustrated in **Fig. 12**. In this computational experiment ASIM generated multiple noisy realizations of a three-dimensional sinogram for whole-body datasets that would be virtually impossible to achieve with MC methods. ASIM is being developed further to provide an integrated environment[72] with the open-source reconstruction package Software for Tomographic Image Reconstruction (STIR),[73] which will enable more efficient four-dimensional simulations and reconstructions of realistic PET data (http://stir.sf.net).

Finally, another demonstration of the powerful capabilities of analytic methods has been recently presented by Tsoumpas and coworkers.[32] This method is used to simulate dynamic PET data based on anatomic and dynamic information from real MR images. After dynamic MR imaging acquisition, fluorodeoxyglucose (FDG) distributions are produced by segmenting four-dimensional MR images and assigning FDG uptake values or, alternatively, using a high-resolution three-dimensional segmented MR

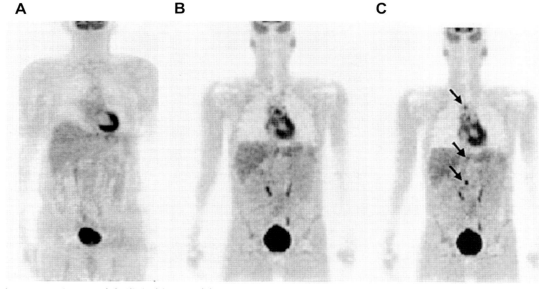

A **B** **C**

Fig. 11. PET images. (*A*) Clinical image. (*B*) PET-SORTEO simulated image of a healthy patient. (*C*) PET-SORTEO simulated pathologic image containing three lesions (*black arrows*). (*From* Tomei S, Reilhac A, Visvikis D, et al. OncoPET_DB: a freely distributed database of realistic simulated whole body 18F-FDG PET images for oncology. IEEE Trans Nucl Sci 2010;57(1):250, http://dx.doi.org/10.1109/TNS.2009.2034375; with permission.)

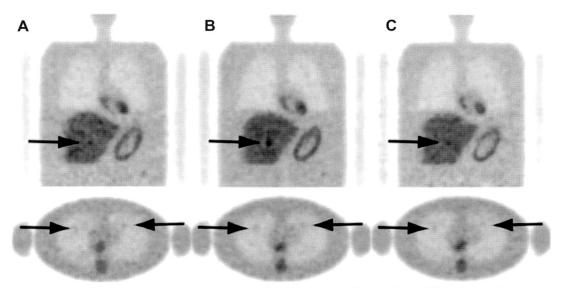

Fig. 12. (*A–C*) Several simulated scans using ASIM software corresponding to three different acquisition protocols. The *arrows* show simulated targets. (*From* Lartizien C, Kinahan PE, Comtat C. A lesion detection observer study comparing 2-dimensional versus fully 3-dimensional whole-body PET imaging protocols. J Nucl Med 2004;45(4):714–23, Fig. 3; with permission.)

image and three-dimensional motion fields from the dynamic MR image. The dynamic FDG distribution is the input to this fast analytic simulation technique (FAST) and raw PET data are created. FAST is performed with a proper combination of STIR utility programs and the simulated projection data include the effects of respiratory motion of the emission and attenuation maps, photon attenuation, and scatter and statistical (Poisson) noise. Realistic four-dimensional simulated datasets[74,75] are freely available to other investigators (http://www.isd.kcl.ac.uk/pet-mri/simulated-data). An example is illustrated in **Fig. 13** and the supplementary animations.[75] An extension of this

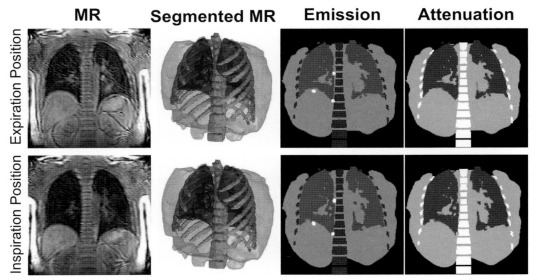

Fig. 13. One plane from expiration (*top row*) and one from inspiration (*bottom row*) positions of the dynamic MR images, and the corresponding derived segmented image; FDG PET distribution; and attenuation image (see also animations). (*From* Buerger C, Tsoumpas C, Aitken A, et al. Investigation of MR-based attenuation correction and motion compensation for hybrid PET/MR. IEEE Trans Nucl Sci http://dx.doi.org/10.1109/TNS.2012.2209127; with permission.)

approach combined real respiratory signal derived from PET-CT images with motion modeling formed from MR imaging acquisitions and used FAST to create almost real-time (100 millisecond) four-dimensional PET simulations. The study investigated the impact of motion blurring on lesion detectability as a function of lesion size, location, and tracer uptake with variable breathing pattern.[76]

FUTURE PERSPECTIVES

Four-dimensional simulations of respiratory and cardiac gated PET acquisitions have made significant progress in the last decade. The availability of multimodal imaging has brought together experts from different radiologic imaging areas and MR imaging and CT data have been used to generate four-dimensional PET data. Although the simulation packages have evolved, more technologic advancements are necessary. There is a need to expand the current simulation toolkits toward a framework that includes irregular respiration patterns and cardiac cycles and bulk motion, peristalsis, and bladder expansion, paving the way toward realistic real-time motion simulations,[77,78] tracer kinetics, and physiologically related motion combined with high-resolution computational phantoms and biologically relevant heterogeneities. These seem to be the future challenges, which once met, will allow more accurate simulation and, consequently, planning and design of PET scanning to the level of complex multicenter clinical trials to improve early diagnosis and therapeutic success.

ACKNOWLEDGMENTS

Dr C. Tsoumpas expresses his gratitude to Dr Christian Buerger for providing the animations and to Professor Paul K. Marsden, Professor Tobias Schaeffter, Dr Volkmar Schulz, Irene Polycarpou, and Dan Balfour for fruitful discussions.

SUPPLEMENTARY DATA

Supplementary data related to this article can be found online at http://dx.doi.org/10.1016/j.cpet. 2012.10.003.

REFERENCES

1. Beyer T, Townsend D, Brun T, et al. A combined PET/CT scanner for clinical oncology. J Nucl Med 2000; 41(8):1369–79.

2. Delso G, Furst S, Jakoby B, et al. Performance measurements of the Siemens mMR integrated whole-body PET/MR scanner. J Nucl Med 2011; 52(12):1914–22.

3. Kalemis A, Delattre B, Heinzer S. Sequential whole-body PET/MR scanner: concept, clinical use, and optimisation after two years in the clinic. The manufacturer's perspective. MAGMA August 7, 2012. http://dx.doi.org/10.1007/s10334-012-0330-y.

4. Zaidi H, Ojha N, Morich M, et al. Design and performance evaluation of a whole-body Ingenuity TF PET-MRI system. Phys Med Biol 2011;56(10):3091–107.

5. Walker MD, Asselin MC, Julyan PJ, et al. Bias in iterative reconstruction of low-statistics PET data: benefits of a resolution model. Phys Med Biol 2011;56(4): 931–49.

6. Chun S, Fessler J. Spatial resolution properties of motion-compensated tomographic image reconstruction methods. IEEE Trans Med Imaging 2012; 31(7):1413–25.

7. Alessio A, Kinahan P. Improved quantitation for PET/CT image reconstruction with system modeling and anatomical priors. Med Phys 2006;33(11):4095–103.

8. Leahy RM, Qi J. Statistical approaches in quantitative positron emission tomography. Stat Comput 2000;10:147–65.

9. Wang G, Qi J. An optimization transfer algorithm for nonlinear parametric image reconstruction from dynamic PET data. IEEE Trans Med Imaging 2012; 31(10):1977–88.

10. Snyder W, Ford M, Warner G, et al. MIRD Pamphlet No. 5: estimates of absorbed fractions for monoenergetic photon sources uniformly distributed in various organs of a heterogeneous phantom. J Nucl Med 1969;10(Suppl 3):7–52.

11. Zaidi H, Tsui BM. Review of computational anthropomorphic anatomical and physiological models. Proc IEEE 2009;97(12):1938–53.

12. Zaidi H, Xu XG. Computational anthropomorphic models of the human anatomy: the path to realistic Monte Carlo modeling in radiological sciences. Annu Rev Biomed Eng 2007;9(1):471–500.

13. Xu X, Chao T, Bozkurt A. VIP-Man: an image-based whole-body adult male model constructed from color photographs of the visible human project for multi-particle Monte Carlo calculations. Health Phys 2000;78(5):476–86.

14. Aristophanous M, Penney BC, Pelizzari C. The development and testing of a digital PET phantom for the evaluation of tumor volume segmentation techniques. Med Phys 2008;35(7):3331–42.

15. Ma Y, Kamber M, Evans AC. 3D simulation of PET brain images using segmented MRI data and positron tomograph characteristics. Comput Med Imaging Graph 1993;17(4–5):365–71.

16. Pollari M, Loetjoenen J, Pauna N, et al. Evaluation of cardiac PET-MRI registration methods using a numerical breathing phantom. In: 2004 IEEE International Symposium on Biomedical Imaging: From Nano To Macro. Arlington (VA): IEEE; 2004. p. 1447–50.

17. Sklyar AV, Gu S, Gennert MA, et al. Generating anthropomorphic phantoms semi-automatically from magnetic resonance images. In: Bo Yu, editor. 2009 IEEE Nuclear Science Symposium and Medical Imaging Conference. Orlando (FL): IEEE; 2009. p. 2743–6.

18. Zubal IG, Harrell CR, Smith EO, et al. Computerized three-dimensional segmented human anatomy. Med Phys 1994;21(2):299–302.

19. Segars WP, Lalush DS, Tsui BM. A realistic spline-based dynamic heart phantom. IEEE Trans Nucl Sci 1999;46(3):503–6.

20. Segars WP, Tsui BM. MCAT to XCAT: the evolution of 4-D computerized phantoms for imaging research. Proc IEEE 2009;97(12):1954–68.

21. Park M, Chen S, Lee T, et al. Generation and evaluation of a simultaneous cardiac and respiratory gated Rb-82 PET simulation. In: Chmeissani M, editor. 2011 IEEE Nuclear Science Symposium and Medical Imaging Conference. Valencia: IEEE; 2011. p. 3327–30.

22. Segars WP, Mahesh M, Beck TJ, et al. Realistic CT simulation using the 4D XCAT phantom. Med Phys 2008;35(8):3800–8.

23. Johnson PB, Whalen SR, Wayson M, et al. Hybrid patient-dependent phantoms covering statistical distributions of body morphometry in the U.S. adult and pediatric population. Proc IEEE 2009;97(12): 2060–75.

24. Segars WP, Sturgeon G, Li X, et al. Patient specific computerized phantoms to estimate dose in pediatric CT. SPIE Medical Imaging 2009;7258: 72580H1–72580H9.

25. Segars WP, Tsui BM, Frey EC, et al. Development of a 4-D digital mouse phantom for molecular imaging research. Mol Imaging Biol 2004;6(3):149–59.

26. Lee C, Lodwick D, Hurtado J, et al. The UF family of reference hybrid phantoms for computational radiation dosimetry. Phys Med Biol 2010;55(2): 339–63.

27. Lee C, Lodwick D, Hasenauer D, et al. Hybrid computational phantoms of the male and female newborn patient: NURBS-based whole-body models. Phys Med Biol 2007;52(12):3309–33.

28. Ruan D, Fessler JA, Balter JM, et al. Exploring breathing pattern irregularity with projection-based method. Med Phys 2006;33(7):2491–9.

29. Martí-Bonmatí L, Graells M, Ronchera-Oms CL. Reduction of peristaltic artifacts on magnetic resonance imaging of the abdomen: a comparative evaluation of three drugs. Abdom Imaging 1996;21(4): 309–13.

30. Button MR, Staffurth JN. Clinical application of image-guided radiotherapy in bladder and prostate cancer. Clin Oncol 2010;22(8):698–706.

31. Segars WP, Lalush DS, Frey EC, et al. Improved dynamic cardiac phantom based on 4D NURBS and tagged MRI. IEEE Trans Nucl Sci 2009;56(5): 2728–38.

32. Tsoumpas C, Buerger C, King AP, et al. Fast generation of 4D PET-MR data from real dynamic MR acquisitions. Phys Med Biol 2011;56(20):6597–613.

33. Buerger C, Schaeffter T, King AP. Hierarchical adaptive local affine registration for fast and robust respiratory motion estimation. Med Image Anal 2011; 15(4):551–64.

34. Chung AJ, Camici PG, Yang GZ. Cardiac PET motion correction using materially constrained transform models. In: Medical imaging and augmented reality, vol. 5128. Berlin: Springer-Verlag; 2008. p. 193–201.

35. King AP, Buerger C, Tsoumpas C, et al. Thoracic respiratory motion estimation from MRI using a statistical model and a 2-D image navigator. Med Image Anal 2011;16(1):252–64.

36. Liu C, Pierce L, Alessio A, et al. The impact of respiratory motion on tumor quantification and delineation in static PET/CT imaging. Phys Med Biol 2009; 54(24):7345–62.

37. McQuaid SJ, Lambrou T, Cunningham VJ, et al. The application of a statistical shape model to diaphragm tracking in respiratory-gated cardiac PET images. Proc IEEE 2009;97(12):2039–52.

38. Schleyer P, O'Doherty M, Barrington S, et al. A comparison of approaches to reduce respiratory motion artifacts in NH3 PET/CT imaging. J Nucl Med 2012;53(Suppl 1):484.

39. Yang Y, Rendig S, Siegel S, et al. Cardiac PET imaging in mice with simultaneous cardiac and respiratory gating. Phys Med Biol 2005;50(13): 2979–89.

40. Fung G, Higuchi T, Park M, et al. Development of a 4D digital phantom for tracer kinetic modeling and analysis of dynamic perfusion PET and SPECT simulation studies. In: Chmeissani M, editor. 2011 IEEE Nuclear Science Symposium and Medical Imaging Conference. Valencia: IEEE; 2011. p. 4192–5.

41. Rosso L, Brock CS, Gallo JM, et al. A new model for prediction of drug distribution in tumor and normal tissues: pharmacokinetics of temozolomide in glioma patients. Cancer Res 2009;69(1):120–7.

42. Rosso L, Gee AD, Gould IR. Ab initio computational study of positron emission tomography ligands interacting with lipid molecule for the prediction of nonspecific binding. J Comput Chem 2008;29(14): 2397–405.

43. Guo Q, Brady M, Gunn RN. A biomathematical modeling approach to central nervous system radioligand discovery and development. J Nucl Med 2009;50(10):1715–23.

44. Guo Q, Owen DR, Rabiner EA, et al. Identifying improved TSPO PET imaging probes through biomathematics: the impact of multiple TSPO binding sites in vivo. Neuroimage 2012;60(2):902–10.

45. Tomasi G, Kimberley S, Rosso L, et al. Double-input compartmental modeling and spectral analysis for the quantification of positron emission tomography data in oncology. Phys Med Biol 2012;57(7):1889–906.

46. Torres Martin de Rosales R, Årstad E, Blower P. Nuclear imaging of molecular processes in cancer. Target Oncol 2009;4(3):183–97.

47. Wessel C, Schnabel JA, Brady M. Towards a more realistic biomechanical modelling of breast malignant tumours. Phys Med Biol 2012;57(3):631–48.

48. Coogan J, Humphrey J, Figueroa C. Computational simulations of hemodynamic changes within thoracic, coronary, and cerebral arteries following early wall remodeling in response to distal aortic coarctation. Biomech Model Mechanobiol 2012. March 14, 2012. http://dx.doi.org/10.1007/s10237-012-0383-x.

49. Xiong G, Figueroa C, Xiao N, et al. Simulation of blood flow in deformable vessels using subject-specific geometry and spatially varying wall properties. Int J Numer Method Biomed Eng 2010;27(7):1000–16.

50. Cookson A, Lee J, Michler C, et al. A novel porous mechanical framework for modelling the interaction between coronary perfusion and myocardial mechanics. J Biomech 2012;45(5):850–5.

51. Nordsletten DA, Niederer SA, Nash MP, et al. Coupling multi-physics models to cardiac mechanics. Prog Biophys Mol Biol 2011;104(1–3):77–88.

52. Smith N, Waters S, Hunter P, et al. The cardiac physiome: foundations and future prospects for mathematical modelling of the heart. Prog Biophys Mol Biol 2011;104(1–3):1.

53. Dubsky S, Hooper S, Siu K, et al. Synchrotron-based dynamic computed tomography of tissue motion for regional lung function measurement. J R Soc Interface 2012;9(74):2213–24.

54. Jan S, Santin G, Strul D, et al. GATE: a simulation toolkit for PET and SPECT. Phys Med Biol 2004;49(19):4543–61.

55. Gonias P, Bertsekas N, Karakatsanis N, et al. Validation of a GATE model for the simulation of the Siemens Biograph 6 PET scanner. Nucl Instrum Methods Phys Res A 2007;571:263–6.

56. Karakatsanis N, Sakellios N, Tsantilas NX, et al. Comparative evaluation of two commercial PET scanners, ECAT EXACT HR+ and Biograph 2, using GATE. Nucl Instrum Methods Phys Res A 2006;569(2):368–72.

57. Lamare F, Turzo A, Bizais Y, et al. Validation of a Monte Carlo simulation of the Philips Allegro/GEMINI PET systems using GATE. Phys Med Biol 2006;51(4):943–62.

58. Lewellen TK, Harrison RL, Vannoy S. "The SimSET program" in Monte Carlo calculations in nuclear medicine. In: Ljungberg M, Strand SE, King MA, editors. Applications in diagnostic imaging. Bristol (England): Institute of Physics Publishing; 1998. p. 77–92.

59. Reilhac A, Batan G, Michel C, et al. PET-SORTEO: validation and development of database of simulated PET volumes. IEEE Trans Nucl Sci 2005; 52(5):1321–8.

60. España S, Herraiz JL, Vicente E, et al. PeneloPET, a Monte Carlo PET simulation tool based on PENELOPE: features and validation. Phys Med Biol 2009;54(6):1723–42.

61. Zaidi H, Labbé C, Morel C. Implementation of an environment for Monte Carlo simulation of fully 3-D position tomography on a high-performance parallel plateform. Parallel Comput 1998;24(9–10):1523–36.

62. Arce P, Rato P, Cañadas M, et al. GAMOS: a Geant4-based easy and flexible framework for nuclear medicine applications. In: Sellin P, editor. 2008 IEEE Nuclear Science Symposium and Medical Imaging Conference. Dresden: IEEE; 2008. p. 3162–8.

63. McLennan A, Reilhac A, Brady M. SORTEO: Monte Carlo-based simulator with list-mode capabilities. 31st Annual International Conference of the IEEE EMBS Minneapolis, Minnesota, USA, September 2–6, 2009. Conf Proc IEEE Eng Med Biol Soc 2009;3751–4.

64. Zaidi H, Scheurer AH, Morel C. An object-oriented Monte Carlo simulator for 3D positron tomographs. Comput Methods Programs Biomed 1999;57(2):133–45.

65. Cañadas M, Arce P, Mendes PR. Validation of a small-animal PET simulation using GAMOS: a GEANT4-based framework. Phys Med Biol 2011;56(1):273–88.

66. Buvat I, Castiglioni I. Monte Carlo simulations in SPET and PET. Q J Nucl Med 2002;46(1):48–61.

67. Tomei S, Reilhac A, Visvikis D, et al. OncoPET_DB: a freely distributed database of realistic simulated whole body 18F-FDG PET images for oncology. IEEE Trans Nucl Sci 2010;57(1):246–55.

68. Le Maitre A, Segars WP, Marache S, et al. Computed data, that describes the anatomy and breathing-motion of individual cancer patients, is used to increase the realism of computer models that represent the patients bodies. Proc IEEE 2009;97(12):2026–38.

69. Ma Y, Evans AC. Analytical modeling of PET imaging with correlated functional and structural images. IEEE Trans Nucl Sci 1997;44(6):2439–44.

70. Comtat C, Kinahan P, Defrise M, et al. Simulating whole-body PET scanning with rapid analytical methods. In: Seibert A, editor. 1999 IEEE Nuclear Science Symposium and Medical Imaging Conference. Seattle (WA): IEEE; 1999. p. 1260–4.

71. Lartizien C, Kinahan PE, Comtat C. A lesion detection observer study comparing 2-dimensional versus

fully 3-dimensional whole-body PET imaging protocols. J Nucl Med 2004;45(4):714–23.

72. Kinahan P, Harisson RL, Elston B, et al. An integrated simulation and reconstruction environment for PET imaging. Presented at the 2012 IEEE Nuclear Science Symposium and Medical Imaging Conference. Anaheim, October 29 to November 3, 2012.

73. Thielemans K, Tsoumpas C, Mustafovic S, et al. STIR: software for tomographic image reconstruction release 2. Phys Med Biol 2012;57(4):867–83.

74. Polycarpou I, Tsoumpas C, Marsden PK. Analysis and comparison of two methods for motion correction in PET imaging. Med Phys 2012; 39(10):6474–83.

75. Buerger C, Tsoumpas C, Aitken A. Investigation of MR-based attenuation correction and motion compensation for hybrid PET/MR. IEEE Trans Nucl Sci 2012;59(5):1967–76.

76. Polycarpou I, Tsoumpas C, Marsden P. Localization ROC Analysis of the impact of respiratory motion correction on lesion detection in PET: a simulation study based on real MR dynamic data. Presented at the 2012 IEEE Nuclear Science Symposium and Medical Imaging Conference. Anaheim, October 29 to November 3, 2012.

77. Churchill N, Chamberland M, Xu T. Algorithm and simulation for real-time positron emission based tumor tracking using a linear fiducial marker. Med Phys 2009;36(5):1576–86.

78. Xu T, Wong J, Shikhaliev P, et al. Real-time tumor tracking using implanted positron emission markers: concept and simulation study. Med Phys 2006;33(7): 2598–609.

Index

Note: Page numbers of article titles are in **boldface** type.

PET Clin 8 (2013) 111–115
http://dx.doi.org/10.1016/S1556-8598(12)00157-5
1556-8598/13/$ – see front matter © 2013 Elsevier Inc. All rights reserved.

pet.theclinics.com

Moving?

Make sure your subscription moves with you!

To notify us of your new address, find your **Clinics Account Number** (located on your mailing label above your name), and contact customer service at:

Email: journalscustomerservice-usa@elsevier.com

800-654-2452 (subscribers in the U.S. & Canada)
314-447-8871 (subscribers outside of the U.S. & Canada)

Fax number: 314-447-8029

Elsevier Health Sciences Division
Subscription Customer Service
3251 Riverport Lane
Maryland Heights, MO 63043

*To ensure uninterrupted delivery of your subscription, please notify us at least 4 weeks in advance of move.